REVIVING YOUR BODY WITH THE ANTI-INFLAMMATORY DIET

Science-Driven Nutrition for Supporting Wellness with Chronic Conditions

A STEP-BY-STEP GUIDE FOR WEIGHT MANAGEMENT NATURALLY

A BONUS QUICK AND EASY ANTI-INFLAMMATORY RECIPE BOOK

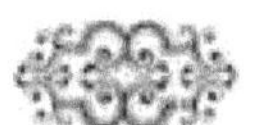

A. A. OLSON

This book is intended as a source of general information on health and wellness and is not a substitute for professional medical advice, diagnosis, or treatment. Always seek the advice of your physician or other qualified health provider with any questions you may have regarding a medical condition or treatment.

First Edition

Printed in the United States of America

Disclaimer: Every effort has been made to ensure the accuracy of the information presented in this book. The author and publisher are not responsible for any adverse effects resulting from the application or use of the information contained herein. Readers are advised to consult with a healthcare professional before making any significant dietary or lifestyle changes.

CONTENTS

Introduction   7

1. Understanding Inflammation   10
   1.1 The Science Of Inflammation   10

   1.2 Chronic Inflammation And Your Health   12

   1.3 Identifying Inflammatory Triggers   14

   1.4 Inflammation Markers: What They Mean For You   16

2. The Anti-Inflammatory Diet Basics   19
   2.1 Personalized Anti-Inflammatory Strategies   21

   2.2 Anti-Inflammatory Superfoods: What To Include   23

   2.3 Debunking Common Diet Myths   25

3. Supplements And Natural Remedies   28
   3.1 Herbal Remedies With Scientific Backing   31

   3.2 Fermented Foods And Gut Health   33

   3.3 Exploring Adaptogens And Their Benefits   34

4. Holistic Approaches To Inflammation   37
   4.1 Exercise For Reducing Inflammation   40

   4.2 The Power Of Sleep In Healing   42

   4.3 Mindful Eating And Its Benefits   43

5. Foods To Embrace And Avoid   46
   5.1 Identifying And Avoiding Inflammatory Foods   48

   5.2 Grocery Shopping With An Anti-Inflammatory Focus   50

   5.3 Snacking Smart On The Go   51

6. Integrating Anti- Inflammatory Living   55
   6.1 Adapting The Diet For Family And Friends   57

6.2 Navigating Holidays And Special Occasions   59

6.3 Sustaining Long-Term Health Benefits   61

7. Addressing Common Pain Points   64
7.1 Craving Reflection Exercise   66

7.2 Eating Out Without Compromising Your Diet   66

7.3 Budget-Friendly Anti-Inflammatory Choices   68

7.4 Overcoming Weight Management Challenges   69

8. Recipes And Culinary Inspiration   72
8.1 Plant-Based Cooking Challenge   74

8.2 Gluten-Free And Dairy-Free Recipes   74

8.3 Incorporating Anti-Inflammatory Spices   76

8.4 International Cuisine With An Anti-Inflammatory Twist   78

9. Practical Meal Planning   80
9.1 Meal Planning For Busy Adults   80

9.2 Batch Cooking And Freezing Anti-Inflammatory Meals   82

9.3 Quick And Easy Breakfasts   84

9.4 Family-Friendly Meal Ideas   85

10. Success Stories   88
10.1 Overcoming Chronic Illness With Diet   90

10.2 Long-Term Health Improvements   92

10.3 Stories Of Weight Management Success   94

11. Tracking Progress And Staying Motivated   95
11.1 Using Technology To Track Your Journey   99

11.2 Celebrating Small Wins   100

11.3 Building A Supportive Community   103

Conclusion 106

Bonus Recipe Book 108
Anti-Inflammatory Meals Under 30 Minutes 108

The Anti-Inflammatory Breakfast 108

Lunch And Dinner Recipes 133

Simple Snacks And Smoothies 200

References 223

INTRODUCTION

One evening, as I settled down for dinner, what lay before me looked more like a war zone than a meal. It was a typical dinner, yet the sensations I experienced were anything but ordinary.

Alongside my meal, I faced persistent joint pain, mental fog, and relentless fatigue—ailments that felt all too familiar. In that moment of discomfort, I realized that my body was sending a crucial warning, a silent protest against the ongoing inflammation within.

As a registered medical professional knowing about the systemic connection, I have spent years studying the intricate connections between the human body and the systemic link. I have been continually learning the effects inflammation can have on your health. My journey began with a simple yet profound question: How can we use food to heal? With a deep commitment to bridging science and practical nutrition, I have dedicated my background and research to helping myself and others understand how diet can be a powerful tool in managing health, particularly when it comes to chronic conditions.

This book's purpose is clear. It seeks to educate you on how an anti-inflammatory diet can transform your health, manage chronic conditions, and support natural weight management. It is not just about what you eat but how those choices impact your body's internal processes.

Inflammation, while a natural immune system response, can become a silent antagonist when it lingers beyond its welcome. Chronic inflammation is linked to numerous ailments, from arthritis to heart disease, and understanding how to manage it is crucial for your well-being.

The concept of inflammation is straightforward yet profound. It is the body's defense mechanism to fight off injury and infection. But when inflammation becomes chronic, it turns from protector to foe. This persistent state can lead to various health issues, affecting your quality of life.

Managing inflammation is not just about alleviating symptoms but addressing the root causes and preventing further harm.

This book is organized into several sections designed to deepen your understanding and application of the anti-inflammatory diet. We begin by exploring inflammation, its causes, and its effects. Next, we delve into the science behind the anti-inflammatory diet, supported by evidence-based research and case studies. Practical meal plans and quick, easy recipes follow, ensuring you can integrate these principles into your daily life. Finally, you'll find success stories and testimonials that illustrate the transformative power of these dietary changes. Chapter 12 delivers your Anti-Inflammatory Cookbook with over 40 recipes. All with visually appealing images. To keep printing costs down and pass the savings onto you, with grey scale images to get the appetites for healthy food moving.

As you read, you can expect to gain a comprehensive understanding of how to reduce inflammation through diet. You'll find practical meal plans that are easy to follow and recipes that fit seamlessly into your busy lifestyle. This book addresses common concerns, such as how to enjoy your favorite foods while still adhering to an anti-inflammatory diet. You'll learn which foods can help with joint pain and how to manage chronic illnesses like arthritis through diet.

Throughout this journey, I'll address your questions, such as identifying inflammatory foods, handling cravings, and staying motivated when progress seems slow. You'll discover the best snacks to support your diet on the go and learn about supplements that can complement your efforts. I offer guidance on effective monitoring to help you track your progress and see the benefits.

This book is more than a guide; it's an invitation to take control of your health journey. With informed dietary choices, you have the power to change your life. I encourage you to embrace this opportunity with open arms, knowing that every small step brings you closer to revitalized health and well-being. Let's embark on this path together, transforming not just meals but entire lives.

CHAPTER 1

UNDERSTANDING INFLAMMATION

As you wake up, your body hums with life, a symphony of biological processes working in harmony. Unseen forces protect and repair you, responding to every cut, bruise, or hint of illness. This is your immune system at work, a vigilant guardian defending against unseen threats. Inflammation is at the heart of this defense, a powerful yet misunderstood player in your body's health narrative. You might wonder why something meant to protect can sometimes cause harm. This chapter will unravel the mysteries of inflammation, providing insight into its dual nature and impact on your well-being.

1.1 THE SCIENCE OF INFLAMMATION

Inflammation, at its core, is the body's response to threats. When you twist an ankle or catch a cold, your body responds with inflammation, marked by redness, swelling, and warmth. This acute inflammation is your body's emergency response, marshaling white blood cells to the site of injury or infection. These cells wage a microscopic battle to isolate and eliminate invaders like bacteria or viruses. You might notice discomfort, but this is a sign that your body is healing. The swelling and pain are reminders of the complex biological choreography beneath your skin, where white blood cells and proteins converge to repair damage and prevent further harm.

Yet, inflammation is not always benign. While acute inflammation is a necessary healing process, chronic inflammation can be destructive. When inflammation persists long after the initial trigger has vanished, it transitions from a helpful friend to a potential foe. Chronic inflammation festers quietly, often without apparent symptoms, slowly damaging tissues and contributing to diseases. This dual nature of inflammation makes it both fascinating and crucial to understand. On one hand, it is a protective mechanism, shielding you from harm. On the other, when unchecked, it can lead to conditions like arthritis, heart disease, and diabetes, silently impacting your health over time.

Recognizing the critical players involved is essential to grasp inflammation's complexity. Cytokines, small proteins released by cells, act as messengers, orchestrating the inflammatory response. They signal other cells to join the battle, ensuring a coordinated defense. Meanwhile, macrophages and neutrophils, white blood cells, act as foot soldiers. Macrophages engulf debris and pathogens, cleaning up the battlefield, while neutrophils rush to the scene, attacking invaders with precision. This intricate dance between cells and molecules enables your body to respond swiftly to threats.

Chronic inflammation is a silent contributor to many diseases. Conditions like arthritis, characterized by inflamed and painful joints, and cardiovascular disease, where inflammation plays a role in plaque buildup in the arteries, highlight its widespread effects. Autoimmune diseases, where the body mistakenly attacks its tissues, often have roots in inflammatory processes gone awry. Digestive issues, like inflammatory bowel disease, highlight the role of inflammation in gut health. Even diabetes, a condition often associated with blood sugar levels, has links to persistent inflammation affecting insulin sensitivity.

Understanding inflammation's role in these common health issues is vital. It underscores the importance of managing inflammation to soothe immediate discomfort and prevent long-term damage. Inflammation, while a necessary biological response, requires balance. Left unchecked, it can transform from a healing force to a catalyst for chronic disease. By exploring the science of inflammation, you gain the knowledge needed to make informed choices about your health. This understanding empowers you to take proactive steps, reducing inflammation through diet and lifestyle changes and ultimately improving your overall well-being.

1.2 CHRONIC INFLAMMATION AND YOUR HEALTH

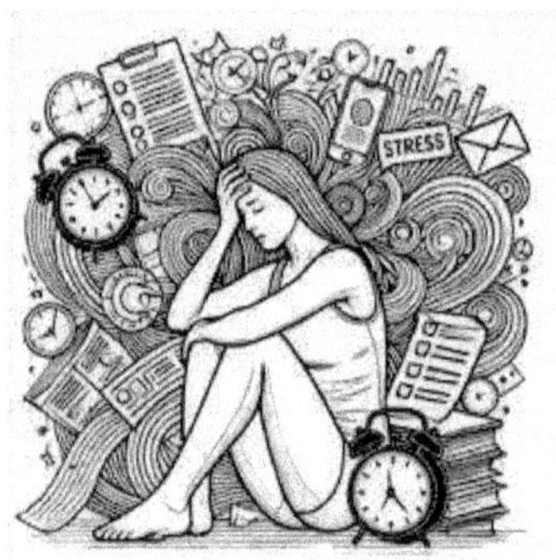

Chronic inflammation is a subtle, persistent inflammation that lingers in the body, often unnoticed. Unlike the immediate and visible signs of acute inflammation, chronic inflammation operates quietly, working beneath the surface. It may not announce itself with swelling or pain, yet its presence is insidious. This low-level inflammation persists, slowly affecting the body's tissues and organs. Factors contributing to chronic inflammation are varied and can include lifestyle choices, environmental exposures, and even long-standing infections. A diet high in processed foods, rich in sugars and unhealthy fats, can fuel inflammation. Likewise, a sedentary lifestyle, where movement is minimal and prolonged periods of inactivity are the norm. Stress also, with chronic stress triggering inflammatory pathways that keep the body in a state of heightened alert. These elements combine, creating a storm of ongoing inflammation that can profoundly affect health.

The implications of chronic inflammation are far-reaching, weaving into the fabric of many severe health conditions. It lays the groundwork for autoimmune disorders, where the immune system mistakenly attacks healthy cells, leading to lupus and rheumatoid arthritis. These conditions manifest through painful symptoms, affecting daily life and overall quality of health. Chronic inflammation also plays a role in metabolic syndrome, a cluster of conditions that include increased blood pressure, high blood sugar, and abnormal cholesterol levels. This syndrome heightens the risk of heart disease, stroke, and type 2 diabetes. Furthermore, chronic inflammation is implicated in neurodegenerative diseases, such as Alzheimer's and Parkinson's, where it contributes to the progressive decline in cognitive and motor functions. As research continues, the links between chronic inflammation and these diseases become increasingly apparent, highlighting the critical need to address and manage inflammation effectively.

Lifestyle is a significant determinant of chronic inflammation, with diet, exercise, and stress management playing pivotal roles. A diet laden with processed foods, such as refined carbohydrates and trans fats, is a significant contributor. These foods trigger inflammatory responses and should be minimized to reduce inflammation. In contrast, diets rich in vegetables, fruits, nuts, and whole grains have been shown to combat inflammation and promote health. Regular physical activity is another antidote to inflammation. Exercise helps maintain a healthy weight and reduces inflammatory markers in the body. Even moderate activity can have substantial anti-inflammatory effects. Stress management is equally vital, as chronic stress can activate inflammatory pathways. Techniques such as mindfulness meditation, deep breathing exercises, and yoga can reduce stress and its inflammatory impact, promoting a more balanced physiological state.

Scientific evidence strongly supports the connection between chronic inflammation and various health conditions. Numerous studies have documented the role of inflammation in disease development, using both observational data and experimental research. For instance, epidemiological studies have highlighted the correlation between elevated inflammatory markers and increased risk of cardiovascular disease, diabetes, and other chronic conditions. These findings are reinforced by research showing that anti-inflammatory diets and lifestyle changes can lower these markers, reducing disease risk and improving health outcomes. The growing body of evidence underscores the importance of addressing chronic inflammation to alleviate symptoms and prevent the onset of more severe health issues.

Understanding chronic inflammation and its impacts is crucial for taking control of your health. Recognizing the factors contributing to inflammation and making informed lifestyle choices can reduce its presence in your life. Managing a diet, incorporating regular physical activity, and practicing stress reduction techniques are practical steps that can make a significant difference. The scientific community continues to explore the intricacies of inflammation, offering new insights and approaches to manage it effectively. As knowledge expands, so do the opportunities for improving health through targeted interventions.

1.3 IDENTIFYING INFLAMMATORY TRIGGERS

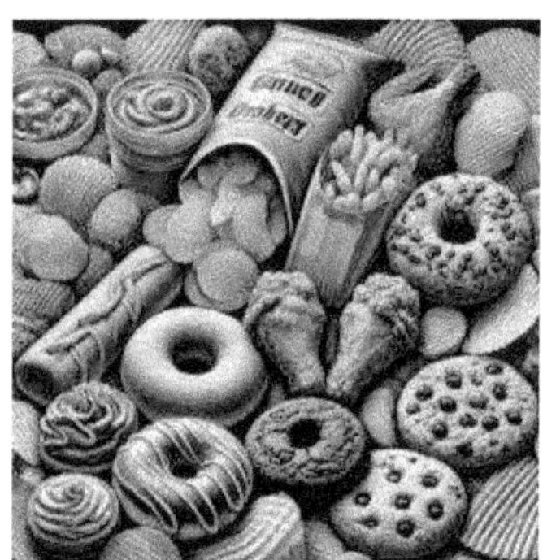

Inflammation, while a complex biological response, often has surprisingly simple triggers, especially concerning diet. One of the most significant instigators found on our plates is processed sugar. This sweet but sinister ingredient lurks in many packaged foods, from cereals to sauces, and it has a knack for stirring up inflammation. Processed sugars can spike insulin levels when consumed, creating a cascade of inflammatory responses affecting various bodily systems. Not far behind are trans fats, often hiding in baked goods and fried foods, which are notorious for their role in promoting inflammation. These fats increase harmful cholesterol levels and contribute to systemic inflammation, making them a double threat. Refined carbohydrates, such as those in white bread and pastries, are also culprits. Stripped of their natural fiber and nutrients, these foods cause rapid spikes in blood sugar, triggering inflammatory pathways that can wreak havoc if consumed regularly.

Beyond diet, our environment and lifestyle choices are pivotal in inflammation. Consider the air we breathe, especially in urban settings where pollutants and toxins abound. These environmental irritants can enter the bloodstream and instigate inflammatory responses, impacting respiratory health and beyond. Stress, another ubiquitous factor, cannot be overlooked. When stress becomes chronic, it triggers the release of stress hormones like cortisol, which can activate inflammatory pathways. This physiological response, meant to be temporary, becomes problematic when sustained, as it can lead to chronic inflammation, affecting mental and physical health. Managing stress through meditation or exercise is crucial to mitigate its inflammatory effects.

Genetics also weave a complex tapestry in the narrative of inflammation. Some individuals may be more predisposed to inflammatory conditions due to genetic markers inherited from their ancestors. These markers can influence how the body responds to various stimuli, making some people more susceptible to inflammation. While we can't change our genetic makeup, understanding these predispositions can inform more personalized approaches to managing inflammation. Knowing your family history and discussing potential genetic influences with a healthcare professional can provide valuable insights into your inflammatory profile and guide tailored strategies for prevention and management.

Identifying personal triggers is paramount to effectively managing inflammation. One practical tool is a food and symptom diary. By documenting daily food intake alongside any symptoms experienced, patterns may emerge that reveal specific dietary triggers. This method encourages mindfulness and can highlight foods that consistently provoke inflammation. Consulting with a healthcare professional can further refine this process. Nutritionists or doctors can provide insights based on medical history and may suggest tests to identify underlying sensitivities or allergies contributing to inflammation.

Additionally, they can offer guidance on crafting a diet that minimizes exposure to known triggers while ensuring nutritional balance. This detective work empowers you to take control of your health. It fosters a deeper understanding of how your body interacts with the world around you, paving the way for informed choices that can significantly reduce inflammation and improve overall well-being.

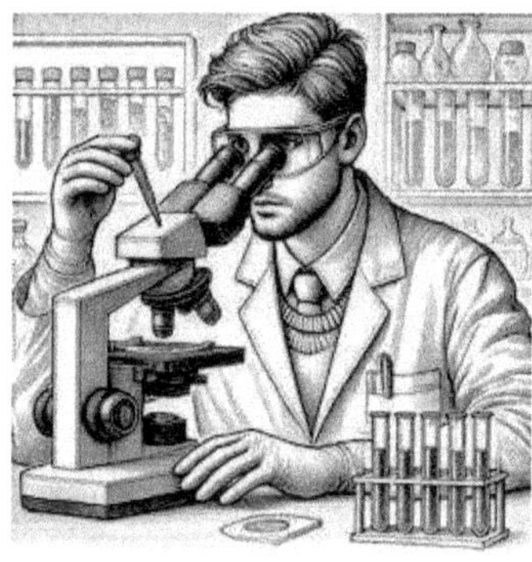

1.4 INFLAMMATION MARKERS: WHAT THEY MEAN FOR YOU

In the realm of health diagnostics, inflammation markers serve a pivotal role. They are the hidden signals of your body's internal state, much like an early warning system.

C-reactive protein (CRP) and erythrocyte sedimentation rate (ESR) stand out. CRP is a substance produced by the liver in response to inflammation. When there is inflammation in the body, CRP levels rise, making it a reliable marker for detecting inflammatory activity.

Similarly, the ESR measures how quickly red blood cells settle at the bottom of a test tube. A faster rate often indicates inflammation. These markers act as vital tools for doctors to gauge the presence and intensity of inflammation, offering insights into potential health issues.

To measure these inflammatory markers, healthcare providers use specific blood tests. For CRP, a blood sample is taken and analyzed to determine the concentration of CRP in the bloodstream. A high level suggests inflammation, possibly due to infection, chronic disease, or other underlying health issues. The ESR test is slightly different. It measures the rate at which red blood cells fall, or sediment, in a tube over an hour. A higher sedimentation rate can indicate inflammation but is not specific to one condition. Instead, it provides a general indication of inflammatory activity, prompting further investigation if needed. While straightforward, these tests offer a window into the body's inflammatory status, helping pinpoint areas of concern.

Monitoring inflammatory markers is not just a one-time affair but a proactive approach to managing health. Tracking these markers can provide valuable information about the body's ongoing inflammatory processes. By observing changes over time, individuals and healthcare providers can detect trends, assess the effectiveness of treatments, and make informed decisions about lifestyle adjustments. For instance, if CRP levels are persistently high, it might be an indication to reassess dietary habits or evaluate stress management practices.

Conversely, decreasing these markers can signal that interventions are working, motivating them to continue on the current path.

When discussing these markers with healthcare providers, preparation is vital. Start by gathering any relevant medical history and documenting any symptoms or changes in health. This information can provide context and help guide the conversation. During the consultation, ask specific questions about what the test results mean and how they relate to your overall health. Understanding the implications of these markers is crucial for making informed decisions about your health. Don't hesitate to seek clarification on any medical jargon or unfamiliar terms. A clear understanding of your test results empowers you to take an active role in managing your health.

For those looking to incorporate inflammation marker monitoring into their health routine, there are several actionable steps to consider. First, consult with your healthcare provider about the appropriateness of these tests for your specific health needs. They can offer guidance on how frequently to test and what levels to aim for. Next, consider lifestyle modifications that can positively impact these markers, such as adopting an anti-inflammatory diet, increasing physical activity, and reducing stress. Finally, keep a record of your test results over time. This can help track progress and identify patterns as a valuable tool in your health management arsenal.

Understanding inflammation markers is a powerful tool in the vast landscape of health and wellness. They offer a glimpse into the body's hidden processes, guiding decisions and shaping strategies for better health outcomes. Individuals can take meaningful steps toward reducing inflammation and improving overall health by engaging with these markers and incorporating their insights into daily life. This proactive approach addresses current health challenges and lays the groundwork for a healthier future, ensuring that the body's internal landscape remains as harmonious as possible. Through informed choices and mindful monitoring, the journey to optimal health becomes a possibility and a reality.

CHAPTER 2

THE ANTI-INFLAMMATORY DIET BASICS

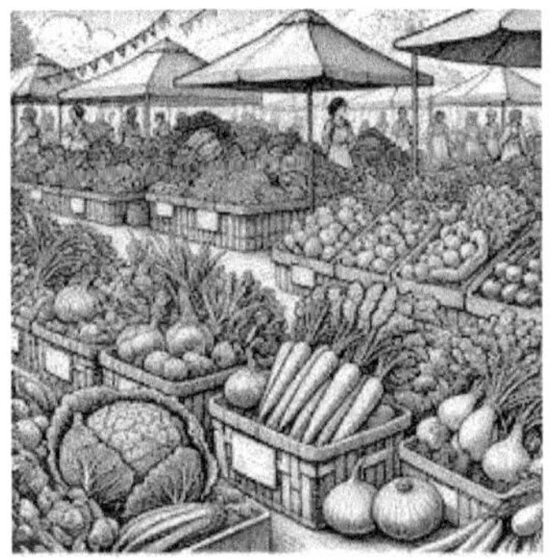

Imagine standing in a bustling market, surrounded by vibrant colors and fresh aromas. Stalls brim with ripe tomatoes, leafy greens, and golden olive oil, each testament to nature's bounty. This vivid scene isn't just a feast for the senses; it's a gateway to health. The choices you make here can profoundly influence your well-being, particularly when it comes to inflammation. This chapter explores the foundational principles of anti-inflammatory eating, a lifestyle that harnesses the power of whole foods to heal and nourish.

The cornerstone of an anti-inflammatory diet is whole, unprocessed foods. Imagine your plate as a canvas, with fresh fruits and vegetables forming the vibrant palette. These foods are rich in antioxidants and fiber, which combat inflammation by neutralizing harmful free radicals and promoting gut health.

Add a handful of spinach to your morning omelet, or toss a medley of colorful vegetables into a hearty stew. Whole grains like quinoa, brown rice, and legumes such as lentils and chickpeas offer complex carbohydrates that provide sustained energy without spiking blood sugar, a key factor in reducing inflammation. By embracing these foods, you lay a solid foundation for health, creating a diet that is as nourishing as delicious.

Healthy fats are pivotal in reducing inflammation and mediating the body's complex biochemical processes. Omega-3 fatty acids found abundantly in fatty fish like salmon and mackerel, are renowned for their anti-inflammatory properties. These essential fats help lower inflammation markers, support heart health, and are linked to improved mental clarity and mood stabilization. Similarly, monounsaturated fats from olive oil and avocados offer protective benefits. Drizzling olive oil over your salad or adding avocado to your sandwich enhances the flavor and fortifies your body's ability to combat inflammation. These fats are integral, working synergistically with other nutrients to optimize your health.

A plant-based focus further amplifies the anti-inflammatory potential of your diet. Leafy greens like kale and Swiss chard are powerhouses of vitamins and minerals. At the same time, cruciferous vegetables like broccoli and Brussels sprouts are rich in compounds that support detoxification and reduce inflammation. By incorporating a variety of these plants into your meals, you reduce inflammation and ensure a diverse intake of nutrients essential for overall health. Consider a simple stir-fry with broccoli and bell peppers or a refreshing salad with mixed greens and cherry tomatoes. These plant-based meals are not just beneficial; they are also versatile and satisfying.

However, limiting processed foods and sugars is crucial, as they can exacerbate inflammation. Processed foods often contain trans fats and added sugars, which are pro-inflammatory and linked to numerous health issues. Reducing your sugary drinks and snacks intake can significantly decrease inflammation levels and improve your overall health. Instead of reaching for a soda, try infusing water with slices of citrus and mint. Replace sugary cereals with oatmeal topped with fresh fruit and nuts. Though seemingly small, these changes can profoundly impact your body's inflammatory state and are essential steps toward sustainable health.

Anti-Inflammatory Shopping List

Create a shopping list focusing on anti-inflammatory foods to guide your next grocery trip. Include:

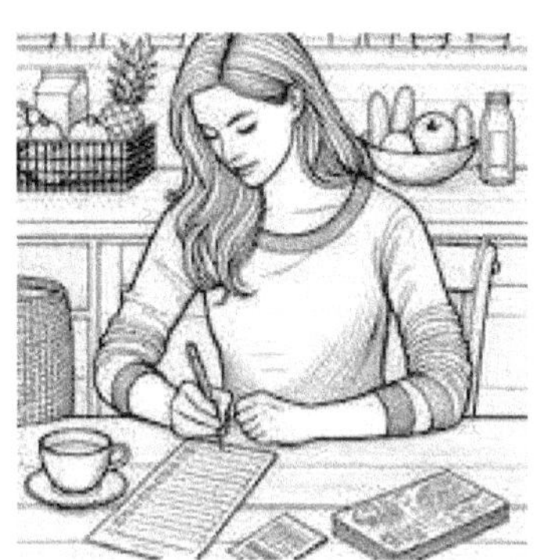

- Fresh fruits and vegetables: Spinach, kale, blueberries, tomatoes, etc.
- Whole grains and legumes: Quinoa, brown rice, lentils, chickpeas.
- Healthy fats include olive oil, avocados, and fatty fish like salmon.
- Herbs and spices: Turmeric, ginger, garlic.

Use this list to plan meals that reduce inflammation and support your well-being.

2.1 PERSONALIZED ANTI-INFLAMMATORY STRATEGIES

Navigating the landscape of dietary changes while managing existing medical conditions can be daunting. You may find yourself at a crossroads, trying to align the anti-inflammatory diet with treatments you are already undergoing. This alignment is essential but requires careful consideration and open communication with healthcare providers. Some may be skeptical, questioning the impact of dietary adjustments on complex health issues. It's essential to approach these conversations with patience and armed with evidence. Present studies and anecdotal success stories that highlight the diet's benefits. This reinforces your commitment to a healthier lifestyle and fosters a collaborative relationship with your medical team. Engaging loved ones in this conversation can be equally challenging. They might harbor doubts about the efficacy of such changes. In these situations, sharing personal goals and the positive changes you've experienced can help bridge these gaps, turning potential resistance into support.

Understanding your nutritional needs is another crucial step. Each body is unique, with dietary requirements influenced by age, activity level, and health conditions. Begin by assessing any food allergies or intolerances requiring specific nutritional adjustments. These considerations are vital in maintaining a diet that reduces inflammation and supports overall health. Balancing macronutrients—proteins, carbohydrates, and fats—based on your lifestyle is equally important. For instance, if you're highly active, you may require more carbohydrates for energy. By aligning your diet with your body's specific needs, you create a plan that is both sustainable and beneficial.

Your cultural background and personal preferences should be noticed. They significantly shape your dietary habits and should be considered when adapting to an anti-inflammatory diet.

Traditional recipes can be modified with anti-inflammatory ingredients, allowing you to maintain cultural connections while promoting health. For example, if your diet is rich in traditional spices or cooking methods, explore how they can be integrated into this new approach. This makes the transition easier and ensures that the diet feels familiar and satisfying. Embracing these personal elements fosters a sense of ownership and enjoyment in your eating habits, making you more likely to stick with the changes.

Flexibility is vital to any successful eating plan. Life is unpredictable, with events and travel often disrupting routine. Creating a flexible eating plan allows you to adapt to these changes without straying from your dietary goals. Consider rotating seasonal foods into your meals, taking advantage of their peak flavors and nutritional benefits. This not only keeps your diet fresh but also supports local agriculture. Planning for special occasions, where indulgence might be tempting, is crucial. Develop strategies to enjoy these events without compromising your dietary principles, such as selecting dishes that align with your goals or bringing your anti-inflammatory options to share.

Regularly monitoring and adjusting your dietary habits is an ongoing process. Keeping a food journal can be an invaluable tool in this endeavor. It helps track what you eat, how it makes you feel, and any changes in inflammation markers. Over time, this record becomes a rich data source, allowing you to identify patterns and make informed adjustments. If certain foods consistently cause discomfort, consider removing them from your diet. Conversely, note any positive changes and reinforce those habits. This approach fosters mindfulness and encourages you to listen to your body's signals, guiding you toward a diet that reduces inflammation and enhances your overall well-being.

2.2 ANTI-INFLAMMATORY SUPERFOODS: WHAT TO INCLUDE

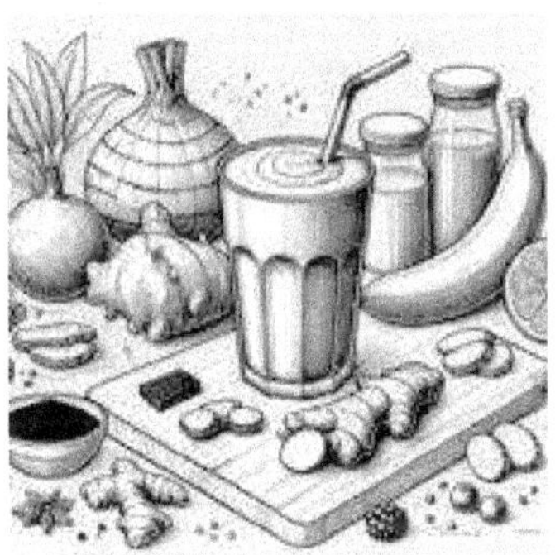

Picture your kitchen counter, a vibrant tableau of nature's finest offerings. There sit blueberries, their deep hue hinting at the rich antioxidants within, ready to combat inflammation and protect your cells from damage. Strawberries join them with their juicy sweetness and high vitamin C content, contributing to lower inflammatory markers in your blood. These berries and other nutrient-dense foods are foundational to an anti-inflammatory diet. Nuts and seeds, like walnuts and flaxseeds, are also essential players. With their omega-3 fatty acids, walnuts and flaxseeds, rich in lignans and fiber, work tirelessly to reduce inflammation and support heart health.

Incorporating these into your diet is as simple as adding a handful to your morning cereal or blending them into a smoothie. They are versatile, easy to use, and pack a powerful punch against inflammation.

Spices, too, hold incredible anti-inflammatory properties, and none are more celebrated than turmeric and ginger. Turmeric, with its active compound curcumin, has been extensively studied for its ability to modulate inflammatory pathways in the body. It can be added to soups, stews, or even roasted vegetables for an earthy flavor and a vibrant pop of color. Ginger, known for its spicy kick, not only adds warmth to dishes but also has compounds that inhibit the production of inflammatory molecules. Brew it in tea or incorporate it into dressings and marinades. These spices are more than just flavor enhancers; they are potent allies in your quest for health.

Dark chocolate, a delightful indulgence, also deserves mention. Its rich antioxidants, specifically flavonoids, have been shown to reduce inflammation and improve heart health. Opt for chocolate with a high cocoa content to maximize these benefits while limiting sugar intake.

Enjoy a small piece as a treat, or melt it into a hot beverage for a comforting and healthful drink. Green tea, another powerhouse, combines polyphenols like catechins that fight inflammation.

Sipping on a cup of green tea can be a soothing ritual supporting your body's defenses. Replace your afternoon coffee with this calming alternative, or use it as a base for smoothies.

Incorporating these superfoods into your daily meals is simpler than you might think. Start your day with a smoothie enriched with chia seeds, which offer omega-3s and fiber, aiding digestion and reducing inflammation. Blend them with berries, spinach, and a splash of almond milk for a nutritious, energizing breakfast. Add turmeric to rice or quinoa when cooking, infusing your grains with anti-inflammatory benefits and a golden hue. These minor adjustments can transform familiar meals into health-boosting powerhouses.

Scientific research underscores the effectiveness of these superfoods. Studies have shown the significant anti-inflammatory effects of omega-3 fatty acids, which are abundant in walnuts and flaxseeds. These studies highlight how regular consumption can lower inflammation markers and reduce the risk of chronic diseases such as heart disease and arthritis. The polyphenols in green tea have been linked to improved heart health and reduced inflammation, making it a wise choice for those seeking to bolster their defenses. Embracing these foods is not just a dietary choice but a scientifically backed strategy for enhancing your health.

As you explore these ingredients, consider how they can be woven into your routines. A bowl of oatmeal topped with berries and a sprinkle of flaxseeds becomes a nourishing breakfast. A lunchtime salad gains depth and nutrition with the addition of walnuts and a ginger-infused dressing. These superfoods are not just ingredients; they are tools for transformation, inviting you to savor each meal with the knowledge that you are nourishing your body and mind. By embracing these superfoods, you are taking decisive steps toward reducing inflammation and improving your overall wellbeing.

2.3 DEBUNKING COMMON DIET MYTHS

In the vast nutrition landscape, few topics are as misunderstood as fats. Many of us grew up hearing that fats were the enemy, responsible for everything from expanding waistlines to clogged arteries. However, it's time to set the record straight. Not all fats are created equal, and some are, in fact, vital for your health. Healthy fats, such as those in avocados, nuts, and olive oil, are crucial to an anti-inflammatory diet. They provide essential fatty acids that support cellular function and help reduce inflammation throughout the body. Conversely, unhealthy fats, like trans fats found in processed snacks and baked goods, contribute to inflammation and should be minimized. So, the next time you drizzle olive oil over your salad or enjoy a handful of almonds, rest assured that these foods nourish you profoundly.

Carbohydrates, another dietary staple, are often at the center of controversy. The rise of low- carb diets has led many to view all carbohydrates with suspicion, yet this oversimplification overlooks complex carbohydrates' role in promoting health. Whole grains, fruits, and vegetables provide your body with fiber, vitamins, and minerals essential for maintaining energy and reducing inflammation. These complex carbohydrates release glucose slowly into the bloodstream, preventing the spikes and crashes associated with refined carbs like white bread and sugary treats. Embracing complex carbohydrates means choosing foods that sustain your energy levels and support your body's natural defenses. It's not about cutting carbs but instead opting for those that fuel your body without inflaming it.

The idea that one diet plan fits all is another myth that deserves debunking. Each person's nutritional needs are unique and shaped by factors such as genetics, lifestyle, and health conditions. While some may thrive on a plant-based regimen, others might find that their bodies respond better to a diet that includes lean meats and dairy. Metabolic differences further complicate the picture, influencing how individuals process and utilize nutrients. Understanding this individuality is vital to crafting a diet that truly works for you. Personalization in diet planning means listening to your body, experimenting with different foods, and paying attention to how they make you feel. It's about building a relationship with your food that honors your unique biology and preferences.

Supplements also enter the conversation with their share of myths. While they can play a supportive role in a well-rounded diet, they are not magic pills. Many believe supplements can replace a balanced diet, but this is far from true. The best way to obtain nutrients is through whole foods, which provide a complex array of vitamins, minerals, and phytonutrients that supplements can't replicate. That said, there are situations where supplements are beneficial. For instance, omega-3 supplements can be helpful for those who don't consume enough fatty fish, and vitamin D supplements might be necessary for individuals with limited sun exposure. It's essential to approach supplements with a discerning eye, understanding their role as a complement to—not a substitute for —a nutritious diet.

As you navigate the world of nutrition, remember that myths and misconceptions abound. Challenge the narratives suggesting fats are inherently bad, carbs are unnecessary, or one diet plan can serve everyone. Embrace the diversity of foods and the unique needs of your body.

Pay attention to how different foods affect you, and be open to adjusting your diet as needed. This mindset empowers you to make informed dietary choices and supports a balanced, inflammation-reducing lifestyle that promotes optimal health. As you move forward, armed with knowledge and curiosity, your journey into the world of anti-inflammatory living continues to unfold, offering new insights and possibilities.

CHAPTER 3

SUPPLEMENTS AND NATURAL REMEDIES

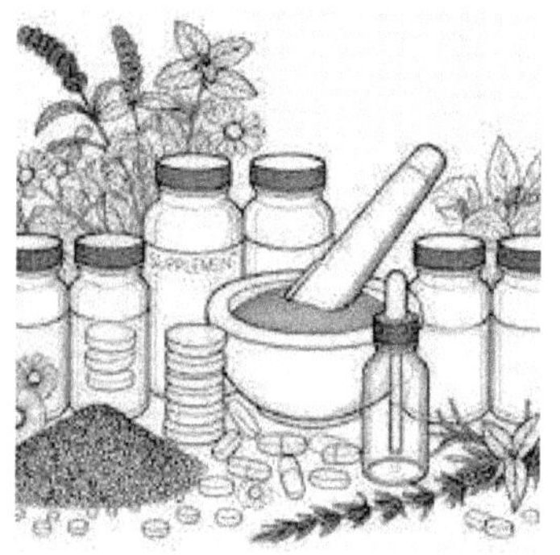

Imagine a symphony orchestra tuning up before a performance. Each instrument, from the violins to the cellos, must be perfectly aligned to create harmonious music. In many ways, your body is similar. It requires a balance of nutrients and supplements to function optimally and maintain health. Certain supplements act like expert musicians when managing inflammation, precisely tuning your body's responses. These supplements can be powerful tools in your health arsenal, helping to reduce inflammation and improve overall well-being.

Omega-3 fatty acids are often hailed as one of the most potent anti-inflammatory supplements. These essential fats, found in fish like salmon and sardines, reduce cytokine production, the proteins that signal inflammation. Research has shown that omega-3s, particularly EPA and DHA, are crucial in preventing heart disease and arthritis by modulating inflammatory pathways. Their benefits extend to brain health, potentially reducing the risk of neurodegenerative diseases. However, it's important to note that the typical Western diet is often deficient in omega-3s, making supplementation a valuable option for many.

Curcumin, the active compound in turmeric, is another formidable supplement for targeting chronic inflammation. Traditional medicine has recognized its anti-inflammatory properties for centuries. Modern science has confirmed its efficacy, with studies showing curcumin's ability to suppress pro-inflammatory pathways and cytokines. Making curcumin a promising therapeutic agent for conditions like arthritis and inflammatory bowel disease. By incorporating curcumin supplements into your routine, you may find relief from inflammation-related symptoms, supporting joint and digestive health.

Vitamin D, often called the "sunshine vitamin," is essential for immune modulation. It plays a pivotal role in regulating the immune system and reducing inflammation. A deficiency in vitamin D can lead to increased susceptibility to infections and inflammatory diseases. Ensuring adequate vitamin D levels through supplementation can help maintain a balanced immune response, promoting overall health. Regular exposure to sunlight and consuming foods rich in vitamin D, such as fortified dairy products, can support these efforts.

When considering supplementing, understanding dosage and safety is crucial. Omega-3 supplements are typically recommended at doses of 250-500 mg of EPA and DHA daily for general health, though higher doses may be needed for specific conditions. Curcumin supplements often require doses of 5002,000 mg per day, depending on the formulation and individual needs. Vitamin D supplementation varies, with recommendations generally ranging from 600-2,000 IU per day, but it's essential to tailor the dosage to individual levels and health goals. Always consult with a healthcare provider before starting any supplement, especially if you are taking other medications, to avoid potential interactions.

Scientific research continues to underscore the efficacy of these supplements. Meta-analyses have highlighted omega-3's effectiveness in reducing inflammation and improving metabolic health, while randomized controlled trials have demonstrated curcumin's potential in managing chronic diseases. These studies provide a strong foundation for incorporating these supplements into your health regimen, offering a natural approach to inflammation management.

Integrating these supplements into your daily routine requires thoughtful planning. For optimal absorption, consider taking omega-3 and curcumin supplements with meals that contain healthy fats. Maintaining a health journal to track supplement intake and any changes in symptoms can also be beneficial. This practice encourages mindfulness and allows you to assess the impact of these supplements on your health. Doing so lets you make informed decisions about your supplementation strategy, adjusting as needed to support your body's balance and well-being.

Supplement Checklist

To help you get started, consider creating a checklist to track your supplement intake. Include:

- Supplement name and dosage
- Time of day taken
- Notable changes in symptoms or energy levels
- Any side effects or interactions

This checklist serves as a practical tool, ensuring consistency and helping you monitor the effectiveness of your supplements.

3.1 HERBAL REMEDIES WITH SCIENTIFIC BACKING

Imagine walking through a lush garden where nature's bounty offers more than just beauty; it provides healing. Among these natural wonders is Boswellia serrata, a resinous tree native to India, celebrated for its potent anti-inflammatory properties. Its active compounds, especially AKBA, help reduce inflammation by blocking an enzyme involved in the process. Making Boswellia a potential treatment for arthritis, as clinical trials have shown it can provide relief. This mechanism helps reduce inflammation, making Boswellia a promising remedy for conditions like arthritis. Clinical trials have shown that Boswellia can relieve pain and improve joint function without the side effects common in many pharmaceutical options. Incorporating Boswellia into your regimen could involve capsules or topical applications, providing a natural alternative for managing inflammation.

Another herbal powerhouse is green tea, renowned not only for its soothing qualities but also for its rich content of catechins. These compounds are powerful antioxidants that combat oxidative stress and inflammation at a cellular level. By neutralizing free radicals, catechins protect cells from damage and support overall health. Green tea's benefits extend to reducing the risk of chronic diseases, including cardiovascular issues and metabolic disorders. Sipping on a cup of green tea daily or using its extract in supplements can effectively harness these anti- inflammatory effects. Consider brewing your tea with fresh leaves to maximize benefits, allowing the catechins to infuse fully.

With its distinctive spicy aroma, ginger is a culinary delight and a remarkable anti-inflammatory agent. Its active compounds, gingerols, and shogaols, inhibit the production of inflammatory cytokines, which promote inflammation, making ginger a valuable ally in managing inflammatory conditions like osteoarthritis. Incorporating ginger into your diet can be as simple as adding fresh slices to boiling water for a refreshing tea or using the powdered form in cooking. Its versatility in sweet and savory dishes means you can enjoy its benefits in numerous ways while supporting your body's natural defenses.

Similarly, rosemary, often found gracing our kitchens, offers more than just flavor. Its extract contains rosmarinic acid, a compound with potent antioxidant properties. By scavenging free radicals, rosemary helps reduce oxidative stress, which is closely linked to inflammation. This herb can be used in cooking to enhance flavors or applied topically as an oil for targeted relief of muscle soreness. Rosemary's dual role as a culinary herb and a therapeutic agent makes it a valuable addition to your routine, providing a simple yet effective means of combating inflammation.

Scientific research continues to validate the efficacy of these herbs in managing inflammation. Clinical trials on Boswellia, for instance, have demonstrated significant improvements in pain relief and joint function among arthritis patients. These studies highlight how Boswellia offers a safe and natural approach to managing inflammatory conditions without the side effects typically associated with conventional treatments. Similarly, green tea's benefits are supported by extensive research linking its catechins to reduced inflammation and improved metabolic health. This growing body of evidence underscores the potential of herbal remedies as viable options in the quest for health and wellness.

Safety and efficacy should be at the top of mind when preparing and using these herbs. Herbal teas are a simple and effective way to incorporate these remedies into your daily routine. For example, brewing a pot of ginger tea or adding rosemary to your marinades can seamlessly integrate these herbs into meals. Tinctures and extracts provide concentrated doses of active compounds, offering convenience and potency. When using tinctures, follow dosage instructions carefully and consult a healthcare professional if you take other medications to avoid adverse interactions. This approach ensures you gain the full benefits of these natural remedies while maintaining safety.

3.2 FERMENTED FOODS AND GUT HEALTH

Imagine your gut as a bustling city populated by trillions of microorganisms that form a complex ecosystem known as the gut microbiome. This microscopic metropolis is pivotal in maintaining your health, influencing everything from digestion to immune function. A balanced microbiome is crucial, as it helps regulate inflammation throughout the body. When gut bacteria are imbalanced, it can lead to systemic inflammation, affecting various bodily systems. This connection between gut health and inflammation underscores the importance of nurturing your microbiome. By fostering a diverse and healthy community of gut bacteria, you can help mitigate inflammation and support overall well-being.

Fermented foods stand out as powerful allies in achieving this balance, acting as natural probiotics that enrich your gut flora. These foods undergo a process of lacto-fermentation, where natural bacteria feed on the sugar and starch in the food, producing lactic acid not only preserves the food but also creates beneficial enzymes and probiotic strains that support gut health. Yogurt and kefir are well-known examples, teeming with live bacteria that aid digestion and contribute to a healthy gut environment. Incorporating these into your diet can enhance your microbiome, promoting a dynamic balance that keeps inflammation in check.

Beyond these dairy options, kimchi and sauerkraut offer plant-based alternatives brimming with probiotics. Kimchi, a staple in Korean cuisine, combines vegetables like cabbage with spices and seasonings, fermenting to develop a rich flavor profile alongside its health benefits.

Similarly, sauerkraut, made from fermented cabbage, is a simple yet potent source of probiotics. These foods diversify your gut bacteria and introduce a range of flavors to your meals. Adding a spoonful of kimchi to your dinner or serving sauerkraut alongside a sandwich can seamlessly integrate these benefits into your daily routine.

Regular consumption of fermented foods offers a multitude of health benefits. One of the most significant is improved digestion, as the probiotics help break down food more efficiently, enhancing nutrient absorption, improving overall digestive health, and reducing issues like bloating and constipation. Moreover, a healthy gut microbiome supports a robust immune response, protecting against pathogens and reducing inflammation. The presence of beneficial bacteria creates a barrier that prevents harmful microbes from taking hold, safeguarding your health. These benefits extend beyond the gut, influencing mood, energy levels, and skin health, making fermented foods a valuable addition to any diet.

Incorporating fermented foods into your meals doesn't have to be complicated. Begin by adding a serving of kimchi or sauerkraut to your plate a few times a week. These can be paired with grains or proteins or even enjoyed on their own as a tangy snack. Miso, a fermented soybean paste, is another versatile option. It can be whisked into soups and dressings, providing a savory depth of flavor while delivering probiotics. For a quick and easy addition, consider kefir smoothies, blending this probiotic-rich drink with fruits and greens for a nutritious start to your day.

Embracing fermented foods means more than just enhancing flavor; it's about fostering a vibrant and resilient gut environment. This approach supports your body's natural ability to regulate inflammation, promoting health from the inside out. As you explore the world of fermentation, you'll discover the culinary delights these foods bring and the profound impact they can have on your well-being. By making these simple yet powerful additions to your diet, you're nurturing your microbiome and empowering your body to thrive in the face of modern-day challenges.

3.3 EXPLORING ADAPTOGENS AND THEIR BENEFITS

Imagine walking through a forest, the air filled with the scent of earthy foliage and the whispers of leaves underfoot. Nature surrounds you with plants that have evolved over millennia to withstand harsh climates and stressors. Among these resilient botanicals are adaptogens, remarkable plant-based compounds that bolster your body's ability to resist stress and reduce inflammation. These natural wonders help maintain balance within the body, enhancing resilience against physical and emotional stressors. Adaptogens work like a thermostat, gently nudging your system toward equilibrium and helping it adapt to external pressures.

A well-known adaptogen is ashwagandha, an ancient herb used in traditional medicine for centuries. This adaptogen is celebrated for its ability to reduce stress and anxiety by modulating cortisol levels, the hormone responsible for stress response. When cortisol levels are balanced, the body can manage stress more effectively, reducing inflammation. Ashwagandha doesn't just calm the mind; it also supports physical stamina and strength, making it a versatile ally in maintaining overall health. Whether in powder form mixed into smoothies or as a supplement, ashwagandha can be a gentle addition to your daily routine.

Rhodiola, another powerful adaptogen, is often associated with enhancing physical endurance and mental clarity, valued for its ability to combat fatigue, increase energy, and improve focus. Rhodiola achieves this by influencing the levels of neurotransmitters in the brain, such as serotonin and dopamine, which are crucial for mood and cognitive function. Athletes and busy professionals can benefit from its properties, which helps them perform better under pressure. Whether facing a demanding project or a long day, Rhodiola can offer the support you need to stay sharp and energized.

Adaptogens offer a range of benefits that extend beyond stress management. They help regulate the immune system, which is closely linked to inflammation. By supporting immune balance, adaptogens reduce the risk of inflammatory responses leading to chronic health issues. Additionally, they promote homeostasis, the body's natural state of equilibrium, which is fundamental for long-term health. Their ability to enhance resilience means that you may find yourself better equipped to handle both physical and emotional challenges over time.

Incorporating adaptogens into your diet requires a thoughtful approach. Adaptogenic teas and tinctures offer a simple way to enjoy these benefits. Brew a calming cup of ashwagandha tea in the evening to wind down, or add a few drops of Rhodiola tincture to your morning beverage for a gentle energy boost. These preparations allow you to incorporate adaptogens into your daily life without drastic changes easily. However, as with any supplement, it's important to seek personalized recommendations from a healthcare provider, especially if you have existing health conditions or take other medications. They can guide you on the appropriate dosages and combinations tailored to your needs.

As you explore the world of adaptogens, consider them part of a broader strategy for health and wellness. They complement other lifestyle practices, such as a balanced diet, regular exercise, and mindfulness, to create a holistic approach to well-being. By integrating adaptogens, you're supporting your body's ability to manage stress and paving the way for improved health outcomes. These plant allies offer a natural, gentle means of enhancing your body's resilience, helping you thrive in today's fast-paced world.

In the next chapter, we will delve into holistic approaches to inflammation, exploring how lifestyle changes, including exercise and mindfulness, can further support your journey toward reducing inflammation and promoting overall wellness. By understanding the multifaceted ways you can support your body, you empower yourself to make informed choices that lead to a healthier, more balanced life.

CHAPTER 4

HOLISTIC APPROACHES TO INFLAMMATION

Imagine standing on a tightrope, carefully balancing above a vast, swirling sea of stress that threatens to engulf you at any moment. This precarious act of balance is one many adults perform daily, often without realizing the toll it takes on the body. Despite being an intangible force, stress manifests naturally, altering your body's chemistry and creating inflammation.

Chronic stress, which lingers and festers, sends continuous signals to your adrenal glands to release cortisol, the hormone often dubbed the "stress hormone." While cortisol plays many roles, including regulating metabolism and immune responses, its prolonged presence can weaken the immune system. Cortisol, in excess, disrupts the body's natural inflammatory response, creating a vicious cycle where stress begets inflammation, and inflammation begets stress.

In this context, managing stress effectively becomes as crucial as managing your diet to reduce inflammation. One of the most accessible tools in your stress-management arsenal is deep breathing. This simple yet effective practice encourages relaxation by slowing the heartbeat and lowering blood pressure. Engaging in slow, deep breaths can activate the body's parasympathetic nervous system, often called the "rest and digest" system, which counters the "fight or flight" response of stress. Progressive muscle relaxation offers another path to tranquility. By systematically tensing and then relaxing different muscle groups, you can achieve a state of physical and mental calm. This technique not only helps in releasing physical tension but also aids in reducing the cognitive load that often accompanies stress.

Time management is another potent strategy in your fight against stress-induced inflammation. By organizing your day and prioritizing tasks, you create a structure that allows for moments of rest and reflection, reducing the chaos that can fuel stress.

Effective time management involves:

- Setting realistic goals.
- Breaking tasks into manageable steps.
- Allowing yourself the grace to adapt when unexpected challenges arise.

This structured approach can help prevent the overwhelm that often leads to chronic stress, thereby mitigating its inflammatory effects.

Mind-body practices such as yoga and meditation are invaluable allies in managing stress. Yoga, combined with physical postures, breath control, and meditation, provides a holistic approach to stress reduction. Certain poses, like Child's Pose or Legs-Up-the-Wall Pose, promote relaxation and help release physical blockages, allowing a free flow of energy and reducing tension. Meditation, on the other hand, focuses the mind and encourages a state of presence and awareness, reducing stress and its impact on the body. Techniques such as mindfulness meditation teach you to observe thoughts and sensations without judgment, fostering a sense of calm and detachment from stressors.

Building a stress-resilient lifestyle involves more than individual practices; it requires creating an environment supporting wellbeing. Establishing a daily routine that incorporates stress-reducing activities can provide stability and predictability, which are essential in managing stress.

Whether it's a morning walk, an afternoon yoga session, or an evening spent journaling, these activities should be non-negotiable parts of your day. Creating a supportive social network is also crucial. Surrounding yourself with friends and family who understand your goals and can offer encouragement and accountability enhances your resilience. This community can become a source of strength, providing comfort and perspective during challenging times.

Consider an interactive element, such as a stress-management checklist, to support your journey further. This tool can help you identify stressors, track stress levels, and incorporate targeted strategies into your daily routine. By checking off each practice and noting its effects, you gain insight into what works best for you and build a personalized roadmap for managing stress.

Stress-Management Checklist

- Identify daily stressors and their sources.
- Incorporate deep breathing exercises.
- Schedule time for progressive muscle relaxation.
- Plan and prioritize daily tasks.
- Set aside time for yoga or meditation.
- Cultivate a supportive social network.
- Reflect on stress levels and adjust strategies accordingly.

Incorporating these holistic approaches into your life can transform how you manage stress and, in turn, reduce inflammation. Addressing stress with comprehensive strategies will pave the way for a healthier, more balanced life.

4.1 EXERCISE FOR REDUCING INFLAMMATION

Picture yourself stepping onto a path that winds through a forest of vibrant green, the air fresh and invigorating. Each step creates a cascade of beneficial reactions within your body, reducing inflammation and promoting overall health. Regular physical activity is a powerful antidote to inflammation, helping to lower levels of inflammatory markers. These markers in your blood that signal inflammation decrease as you exercise consistently. This reduction occurs because exercise enhances blood flow, delivering nutrients more efficiently to tissues and organs.

Improved circulation not only nourishes muscles but also aids in the removal of waste products that can contribute to inflammation. As your heart beats steadily, you actively support your body's natural defenses against chronic inflammation.

Among the various exercises available, some stand out for their anti-inflammatory benefits.

Low-impact activities, such as swimming and cycling, provide excellent options for those seeking to minimize joint stress while still reaping the rewards of physical movement. Swimming offers a full-body workout, buoyed by water's support, allowing for fluid motion that strengthens muscles without undue strain. Cycling, whether on a stationary bike or a scenic trail, engages large muscle groups and boosts cardiovascular health while being gentle on the joints. These exercises offer a balance of intensity and ease, making them suitable for individuals at various fitness levels.

Meanwhile, strength training emerges as another valuable ally. Strength training helps stabilize the body and reduce stress on inflammatory sites by building muscle and supporting joints.

Incorporating exercises such as resistance band workouts or bodyweight exercises can foster resilience and improve overall function.

Specific guidelines are essential to ensure your exercise regimen is effective and safe, particularly if you have chronic inflammation. Begin each session with a proper warm-up, gently preparing your muscles and joints for activity, reducing the risk of injury and enhancing performance. Follow each workout with a cool-down period, allowing your heart rate to return to resting levels and promoting recovery gradually. Listening to your body is vital; it communicates through sensations of fatigue or discomfort, signaling when to ease back or modify activities.

Avoiding overexertion is crucial, as pushing beyond your limits can exacerbate inflammation rather than alleviate it. By respecting your body's cues, you create a sustainable exercise routine that enhances well-being without inviting injury.

Incorporating movement into your daily life doesn't always require a dedicated gym session or structured class. Small, intentional changes can accumulate into significant benefits. Take regular walking breaks to stretch and invigorate your body during work hours. These brief pauses refresh your mind and combat the sedentary lifestyle that can contribute to inflammation. Opt for stairs over elevators whenever possible, using the opportunity to engage your leg muscles and increase circulation. Meetings, often synonymous with sitting, can be transformed into dynamic interactions by standing or walking as you discuss ideas. These adaptations integrate movement seamlessly into your routine, fostering a more active lifestyle.

As you explore these methods of incorporating exercise, remember that consistency is key. Sustainable, regular activity yields the most significant benefits over time. Whether you're drawn to the tranquility of swimming, the rhythm of cycling, or the empowerment of strength training, the important thing is to find activities you enjoy and can maintain. This enjoyment becomes a motivator, ensuring exercise remains a fulfilling part of your life. By weaving movement into the fabric of your day, you combat inflammation and enhance your physical and mental health, creating a foundation for long-term vitality.

4.2 THE POWER OF SLEEP IN HEALING

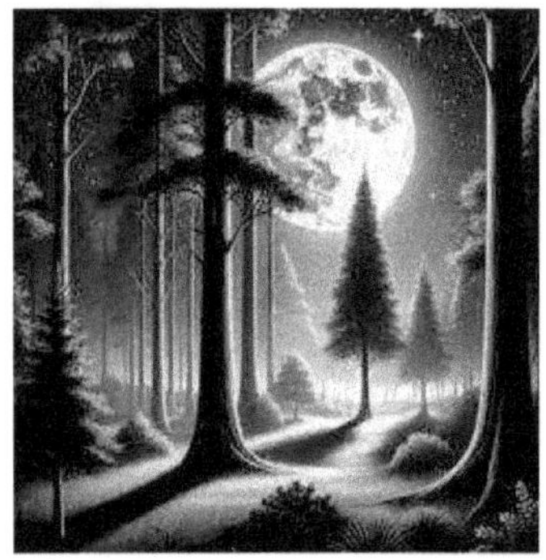

Imagine the quiet of the night when your body enters its most vital state. Sleep is not just a passive activity; it's a dynamic process crucial in managing inflammation and supporting your overall health. During sleep, your body undergoes critical maintenance, repairing tissues and strengthening the immune system. Quality sleep enhances immune function, equipping your body to fend off infections and reduce inflammation. However, a lack of restful sleep disrupts these processes, leading to increased levels of inflammatory markers. This connection between sleep deprivation and inflammation is well-documented, with studies showing that inadequate sleep can elevate levels of cytokines, the proteins that mediate inflammation, creating a state of chronic low-grade inflammation that quietly undermines health over time.

To cultivate an environment conducive to restful sleep, consider the principles of good sleep hygiene. Establishing a consistent sleep schedule is foundational. Going to bed and waking up at the same time each day regulates your body's internal clock, making it easier to fall asleep and wake up naturally. Reducing screen time before bed is another pivotal step. The blue light emitted by phones, tablets, and computers interferes with the production of melatonin, the hormone that regulates sleep. Avoiding screens at least an hour before bed can help your body produce melatonin naturally, signaling it's time to wind down. Creating a calming bedtime ritual further reinforces the transition from wakefulness to sleep. Whether reading a book, taking a warm bath, or practicing gentle stretches, these activities cue your body to relax and prepare for rest.

Poor sleep can have far-reaching effects on your health beyond just feeling tired. Consistently inadequate sleep increases the risk of chronic diseases such as obesity, diabetes, and heart disease. Poor sleep contributes to metabolic dysregulation, increased appetite, and altered glucose metabolism, all of which can exacerbate inflammation. Cognitive and physical performance also suffer, with impaired memory, slower reaction times, and decreased alertness becoming common issues. These effects underscore why prioritizing sleep is not a luxury but a necessity for maintaining optimal health and reducing inflammation.

If you find yourself struggling with sleep disturbances, there are several strategies you can employ to improve sleep quality. White noise machines or earplugs can create a quiet environment conducive to uninterrupted sleep, masking disruptive sounds like traffic or noisy neighbors. Herbal teas, such as chamomile, offer a natural way to promote relaxation and ease the transition to sleep. The calming herb chamomile tea can soothe the nervous system, preparing your mind and body for rest. Maintaining a comfortable room temperature and ensuring your bed is supportive can significantly improve your sleep quality. Adjusting these environmental factors can create a sanctuary where restorative sleep becomes the norm.

Incorporating these strategies into your nightly routine enhances sleep quality and sets the stage for better health outcomes. As you experience the benefits of improved sleep, such as increased energy, sharper focus, and a more balanced mood, you'll find that managing inflammation becomes a natural extension of these positive changes. By valuing sleep and making it a priority, you empower your body to heal and thrive, warding off the insidious effects of chronic inflammation.

4.3 MINDFUL EATING AND ITS BENEFITS

Picture yourself seated at a table, a plate of colorful, nourishing food before you. The room is calm, free from distractions, inviting you to focus intently on the meal in front of you. This is the essence of mindful eating, a practice that encourages you to bring full awareness and intention to eating. Unlike the hurried, often distracted eating habits many of us have fallen into, mindful eating asks you to slow down, savor each bite, and engage with your food on a deeper level. It's about being present in the moment, tuning in to your meal's flavors, textures, and aromas. This approach contrasts sharply with mindless eating, where meals are consumed quickly, often in front of screens, with little thought about the experience. Bringing mindfulness to your meals opens the door to a more harmonious relationship with food that supports your physical and emotional well-being.

The benefits of mindful eating extend far beyond the dining table. Slowing down and paying attention to how and what you eat can significantly reduce inflammation and foster a healthier connection with food. When you eat mindfully, you allow your digestive system the time to properly break down food, leading to improved digestion and more efficient nutrient absorption. Mindful eating helps to alleviate digestive discomfort and ensure your body receives the nourishment it needs. Additionally, mindful eating encourages you to listen to your body's hunger and fullness cues, which can prevent overeating and help maintain a healthy weight. As you become more attuned to these signals, you may feel more satisfied with smaller portions, reducing the tendency to overeat. This supports healthy digestion and helps manage inflammation, as overeating can strain the digestive system and contribute to inflammatory responses.

Incorporating mindfulness into your meals doesn't require drastic changes; instead, it involves subtle shifts in how you approach eating. Begin by taking the time to chew each bite thoroughly, allowing the flavors to unfold on your palate. Eating more slowly not only aids digestion but also enhances your enjoyment of the meal. Engage all your senses as you eat—notice the colors and textures of your food, listen to the sounds of your meal as you prepare and eat it, and savor the aromas that waft from your plate. These sensory experiences can transform a routine meal into a delightful ritual, grounding you in the present moment and deepening your appreciation for the nourishment before you. As you practice these techniques, you may find that your relationship with food becomes more intentional and fulfilling.

Cultivating a mindful eating mindset involves creating an environment that supports this practice. Set aside dedicated meal times to eat without distractions, allowing you to focus on your food thoroughly. This might mean turning off the TV, putting away your phone, and creating a peaceful space for dining. As you eat, take the time to reflect on your hunger and fullness cues, checking in with your body to determine how much food it truly needs. This practice helps you become more aware of your body's signals, encouraging you to eat in a way that honors its needs. By prioritizing mindfulness in your eating habits, you foster a balanced approach to food that supports your physical and emotional wellbeing.

Together, these strategies offer a path to reducing inflammation through mindful eating. By approaching meals with intention and awareness, you create a foundation for a healthier, more satisfying relationship with food. This chapter emphasizes that mindful eating is not just about what you consume but how you engage with the act of eating. As you cultivate this practice, you may find that it extends beyond the table, influencing other areas of your life and promoting a sense of balance and well-being. These holistic approaches to inflammation provide a framework for fully supporting your health, setting the stage for the next exploration of inflammation management.

CHAPTER 5

FOODS TO EMBRACE AND AVOID

Imagine a symphony where each note and instrument works harmoniously, creating a melody that resonates with the soul. Your body functions similarly, relying on a harmonious interplay of nutrients to maintain health, especially when supporting your joints. Just as a conductor guides the orchestra to achieve balance, your dietary choices can orchestrate a symphony of health by nurturing your joints and reducing inflammation. The foods you consume are crucial in maintaining joint health, offering essential nutrients that alleviate pain and bolster overall well- being.

Diet impacts joint health significantly, with certain foods offering a twofold benefit: they reduce inflammation and provide crucial nutrients. Omega-3 fatty acids found abundantly in salmon and flaxseeds, are celebrated for their ability to decrease inflammation. These healthy fats work by inhibiting the production of inflammatory molecules, thus relieving joint pain and stiffness.

Regularly incorporating salmon into your meals, perhaps through a simple grilled fillet with a squeeze of lemon, can make a noticeable difference in how your joints feel. Flaxseeds, on the other hand, are versatile and can be easily added to smoothies or sprinkled over salads, providing a plant-based source of these essential fats. Alongside these, foods rich in antioxidants, such as spinach and kale, play a vital role. These leafy greens are packed with vitamins and minerals that help protect joint tissues from damage, reinforcing the body's defenses against oxidative stress.

Nutrients like vitamin C and collagen are indispensable for joint health. Vitamin C, abundant in citrus fruits, is crucial for collagen synthesis. Collagen is a protein that forms the building blocks of cartilage, the cushioning tissue that protects joints. Consuming oranges, grapefruits, or strawberries can ensure your body has the vitamin C necessary to support collagen production. Similarly, bone broth, a rich source of collagen, provides the amino acids needed to maintain and repair joint tissues. A warm cup of bone broth can be a soothing addition to your diet, offering nourishment beyond mere hydration.

In your quest for joint-friendly foods, cherries are a potent anti-inflammatory option. These vibrant fruits contain anthocyanins, compounds that help reduce inflammation and pain. Enjoy a handful of cherries as a snack, or add them to a yogurt parfait for a delicious and healthful treat. Nuts and seeds also deserve a place on your list. Almonds, walnuts, and sunflower seeds provide healthy fats and antioxidants, contributing to joint health. They can be incorporated into homemade trail mixes or used as toppings for oatmeal and salads.

Consider meal ideas that naturally incorporate these joint-supporting foods. A dinner of grilled salmon and a medley of roasted vegetables, such as bell peppers, zucchini, and carrots, offers a flavorful and nutrient-rich option. Drizzle the vegetables with a touch of olive oil and sprinkle with herbs like rosemary or thyme for added anti-inflammatory benefits. A spinach and berry salad with walnuts can be refreshing and satisfying for a lighter meal. Toss in some sliced strawberries or blueberries, which are rich in vitamin C and antioxidants, and dress the salad with a tangy balsamic vinaigrette.

Focusing on these foods nourishes your body and actively supports your joint health. Each meal becomes an opportunity to reduce inflammation and enhance vitality, transforming everyday eating into a proactive step toward well-being. This approach empowers you to make informed dietary choices, fostering a lifestyle that harmonizes with your body's needs and promotes long-term health.

5.1 IDENTIFYING AND AVOIDING INFLAMMATORY FOODS

Picture a bustling city street where traffic signals control the flow of cars, sometimes leading to smooth travel and other times to frustrating gridlocks. Much like these signals, the foods you consume can direct your body's inflammatory responses, either soothing or exacerbating them. Understanding how certain foods trigger inflammation is crucial in navigating this complex landscape. High-glycemic foods, such as white bread and sugary cereals, cause rapid spikes in blood sugar levels. This sudden influx of glucose prompts the pancreas to release insulin, which can activate inflammatory pathways. Over time, these spikes can contribute to chronic inflammation, much like traffic congestion that slowly wears down a city's infrastructure.

Similarly, trans fats—often lurking in fried and processed foods— disrupt cellular function. These fats raise LDL cholesterol levels and promote inflammation within fat tissue, setting the stage for various health issues.

In the quest for reducing inflammation, it's crucial to be aware of common dietary culprits. Refined sugars and artificial sweeteners top the list, as they are often found in everything from soft drinks to packaged snacks. These sugars trigger the release of cytokines, molecules that can exacerbate inflammation. Another group to watch is processed meats laden with sodium and preservatives. The high salt and chemicals in these meats can irritate the body's tissues, leading to increased inflammatory responses. By recognizing these foods, you can begin to eliminate them and choose healthier alternatives that support your body's natural balance.

Reading food labels becomes an invaluable skill in this endeavor. Labels are like roadmaps, guiding you through the maze of ingredients to identify those that may ignite inflammation. Start by scanning for hidden sugars, which often appear under names like high-fructose corn syrup or dextrose. Unhealthy fats, particularly trans fats, may be listed as partially hydrogenated oils.

Additives and preservatives, while sometimes necessary for shelf life, often contribute to inflammation. Look for natural products with minimal processing to avoid these hidden pitfalls. Understanding these labels means you're not just a passive consumer but an informed participant in your health.

Reducing your intake of inflammatory foods doesn't require a drastic overhaul; small, intentional changes can have a profound impact. Cooking at home with fresh ingredients provides control over what goes into your meals. This practice allows you to select whole foods, free from the excess sugars and unhealthy fats often found in restaurant dishes. Swapping refined grains for whole grains is another practical strategy. Whole grains, like brown rice and quinoa, offer fiber and nutrients that support digestion and reduce inflammation. These changes, though modest, pave the way for a healthier and more balanced lifestyle.

In this journey, the kitchen becomes your ally. Preparing meals from scratch allows you to experiment with flavors and ensures your body receives nourishing, anti-inflammatory foods. Consider creating a weekly meal plan, focusing on recipes highlighting fresh produce and lean proteins. This plan can serve as a guide, helping you confidently navigate grocery aisles. As you become more accustomed to reading labels and making thoughtful choices, you'll find that avoiding inflammatory foods becomes second nature. Much like a well-tuned vehicle, your body will run more smoothly, with fewer interruptions from inflammation.

5.2 GROCERY SHOPPING WITH AN ANTI-INFLAMMATORY FOCUS

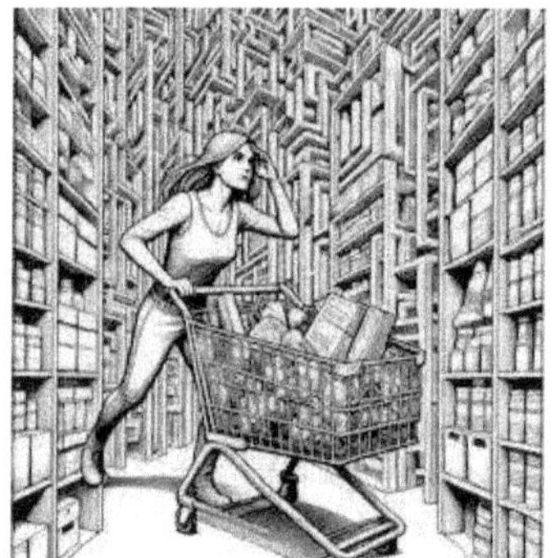

Stepping into a grocery store can feel like entering a labyrinth, with aisles of options vying for your attention. To navigate this maze effectively and prioritize anti-inflammatory foods, start with a well-structured shopping list. This list is your guiding star, helping you stay focused and avoid impulse purchases that may not align with your health goals. Begin by categorizing your list into sections: fresh produce, proteins, and pantry staples. A well-organized list streamlines your shopping experience and ensures you cover all essential food groups. Planning meals ahead of time can further refine your list, allowing you to select ingredients that complement one another and contribute to a balanced diet. This foresight saves time and reduces the temptation to stray from your dietary objectives.

As you traverse the grocery store, focus on the perimeter, where fresh items typically reside. Here, you'll find an abundance of fruits, vegetables, lean proteins, and dairy products. These sections are gold mines for anti-inflammatory options, offering whole, minimally processed foods that are nourishing and sustaining. Conversely, avoiding the inner aisles is wise, as they often house processed and packaged foods loaded with additives and preservatives. By steering your cart toward the store's outer edges, you naturally gravitate toward healthier choices, making it easier to maintain an anti-inflammatory diet. This strategic approach simplifies decision-making and reinforces positive habits over time.

Spotting anti-inflammatory products requires a keen eye and a bit of label literacy. Products labeled as organic or non-GMO can be good quality indicators, but it's crucial to delve deeper. Avoid items with minimal ingredients, avoiding added sugars or artificial preservatives. Foods with short, recognizable ingredient lists are generally better choices, as they are less likely to contain inflammatory additives. For instance, when choosing nut butters, opt for those that list only nuts and perhaps a pinch of salt, eschewing those with hydrogenated oils or sweeteners. By honing your ability to identify these products, you empower yourself to make informed choices that align with your health goals.

Budgeting for anti-inflammatory foods doesn't have to be daunting. There are several strategies to keep costs in check while still prioritizing health. Purchasing seasonal produce is a smart move, as fruits and vegetables in season are often more affordable and flavorful. These items are typically harvested at peak ripeness, ensuring optimal nutrient content. Additionally, taking advantage of coupons and store discounts can significantly reduce your grocery bill. Many stores offer loyalty programs or weekly promotions that provide savings on fresh foods.

Planning your shopping trips around these deals allows you to stock up on nutritious items without straining your budget. These tactics will enable you to embrace an anti-inflammatory lifestyle while remaining financially savvy.

5.3 SNACKING SMART ON THE GO

Maintaining energy levels and reducing inflammation throughout the day can be challenging in a world that never seems to slow down. That's where smart snacking comes into play. Healthy snacks are like mini-meals that fuel your body between the main events, keeping you energized and focused. Yet, choosing the right snacks isn't just about quelling hunger; it's about balancing macronutrients to provide sustained energy. A well-chosen snack should include a mix of carbohydrates, proteins, and healthy fats. This trio works together to stabilize blood sugar levels, curb cravings, and help you feel full longer. Incorporating fiber and protein can be particularly beneficial, as they slow digestion and prolong satiety. Think of snacks as an opportunity to nourish your body, not just fill it.

For those constantly on the move, convenience is key. Portable snack options that align with an anti-inflammatory diet are possible and plentiful. Consider a mix of almonds and dried fruit. This combination offers heart-healthy fats, protein, and natural sweetness without added sugars. The dried fruit provides a quick energy boost, while the almonds keep you satisfied. Veggie sticks paired with hummus are another excellent choice. Cut carrots, celery, and bell peppers into sticks and dip them into a creamy hummus rich in fiber and protein. This snack is easy to prepare, easy to pack, and packed with nutrients. These snacks are convenient and support a balanced diet without sacrificing taste or nutrition.

Preparation is your ally when it comes to healthy snacking. Setting aside a few minutes to prepare snacks in advance can make a world of difference. Portion nuts and seeds into small bags to avoid the temptation of overindulging. These can be stored in your car, office, or backpack, ensuring you always have a healthy option on hand. Another strategy is to make homemade energy bars. You can create delicious bars tailored to your dietary needs using oats, nuts, seeds, and a touch of honey or maple syrup. Once prepared, these bars can be stored in the freezer and grabbed on your way out the door, making them a perfect snack for busy days.

Traveling can present challenges, but with some planning, you can easily navigate these situations. Opt for fresh fruit over packaged snacks when you're on the road. Fruits like apples or bananas are portable and provide quick, wholesome energy. Many convenience stores also offer yogurt cups or hard-boiled eggs, which are excellent protein sources. These practical options align with an anti-inflammatory diet, helping you maintain your health goals even when away from home. Making conscious choices allows you to enjoy travel without compromising your dietary principles.

As you incorporate these snacking strategies, remember that the goal is to support your body's needs throughout the day. Each snack is an opportunity to nourish, energize, and reduce inflammation. By choosing wisely and preparing ahead, you maintain your energy levels and contribute to your long-term health. This approach to snacking becomes a seamless part of your daily routine, empowering you to make choices that align with your health goals. As you continue to explore how diet influences health, you'll find that these simple changes can have profound effects. Whether at home, at work, or on the go, smart snacking is a powerful tool in your wellness toolkit.

A SIMPLE WAY TO MAKE A DIFFERENCE

YOUR REVIEW COULD HELP TRANSFORM LIVES

"The best way to find yourself is to lose yourself in the service of others."

— *MAHATMA GANDHI*

People who give without expecting anything in return live happier lives. So, let's make a difference together!

Would you help someone just like you—curious about living well with chronic conditions but unsure where to begin?

My mission with Reviving Your Body with the Anti-Inflammatory Diet is to make science-backed nutrition accessible, simple, and enjoyable for everyone. I want to help people find balance in their health journeys and rediscover joy in nourishing their bodies.

But to reach more people, I need your help.

Most of us choose books based on reviews. That's why I'm asking you to help a fellow reader by sharing your thoughts. It costs nothing and takes only a moment, but your review could inspire someone to take the first step toward better health. Your words could help…

One more parent provide healthy meals for their family. One more person find relief from chronic discomfort.

One more reader embrace their health journey with confidence.

One more dream of wellness come true.

To make a difference, simply scan the QR code below to leave your review:

CHAPTER 6

INTEGRATING ANTI-INFLAMMATORY LIVING

Imagine your life as a finely tuned orchestra, where each aspect is crucial in creating a harmonious symphony of health. The key to this balance lies in integrating anti-inflammatory practices into everyday life without feeling bound by rigid rules. Instead, it's about embracing a lifestyle that naturally supports well-being, where diverse foods, activities, and moments of mindfulness blend seamlessly into your daily routine. As you embark on this path, consider that balance isn't about perfection but creating a sustainable and nourishing rhythm.

A balanced anti-inflammatory lifestyle begins with variety. Think of your diet as a colorful palette, each meal an opportunity to incorporate a diverse array of foods that provide essential nutrients. Whole grains, lean proteins, and abundant fruits and vegetables should be the mainstays of your diet, each contributing different benefits to your body's health. This variety not only reduces inflammation but also keeps meals exciting and flavorsome.

Alongside this, balance work, leisure, and wellness to create a holistic approach to health. Ensuring that you carve out time for leisure and relaxation is vital, as it provides the space needed to recharge and prevent burnout. This balance allows you to engage fully in each aspect of life, from professional commitments to personal passions, without feeling overwhelmed.

Incorporating anti-inflammatory habits into daily life requires intentionality. Start with morning rituals that set a positive tone for the day. Begin with gentle stretching to awaken your body and promote circulation, followed by a hydrating glass of water infused with lemon or cucumber to kickstart your metabolism. These small acts of self-care can profoundly impact your overall mood and energy levels. Weekly planning sessions for meals and activities can also be a game- changer. You create a framework that supports your anti-inflammatory goals by dedicating a specific weekly time to plan menus and schedule workouts or relaxation exercises. This preparation helps you make informed choices, reducing stress and enhancing your ability to maintain a balanced lifestyle.

Mindfulness is a powerful tool in this journey, offering a pathway to awareness and presence. Practicing mindfulness encourages you to engage with your thoughts and feelings without judgment, fostering a sense of peace and clarity. Incorporate gratitude and positive affirmations into your routine to cultivate a mindset of appreciation and optimism. This practice can be as simple as jotting down three things you're grateful for each day or reciting affirmations that resonate with your personal goals. These practices enhance emotional well-being and provide a buffer against the stressors that can trigger inflammation.

Continuous learning and adaptation are cornerstones of a successful anti-inflammatory lifestyle. The world of nutrition and wellness is ever-evolving, and staying informed empowers you to make choices that align with the latest insights. Dedicate time to reading about new research in nutrition and health and exploring studies that deepen your understanding of how diet and lifestyle impact inflammation. Attending workshops and seminars can also provide valuable knowledge and inspiration, offering opportunities to learn from experts and engage with a community of likeminded individuals. This commitment to learning ensures that your approach remains dynamic and practical, allowing you to adapt practices as your needs and circumstances change.

Reflection Section

Take a moment to reflect on areas of your life where you can integrate balance. Consider the following prompts:

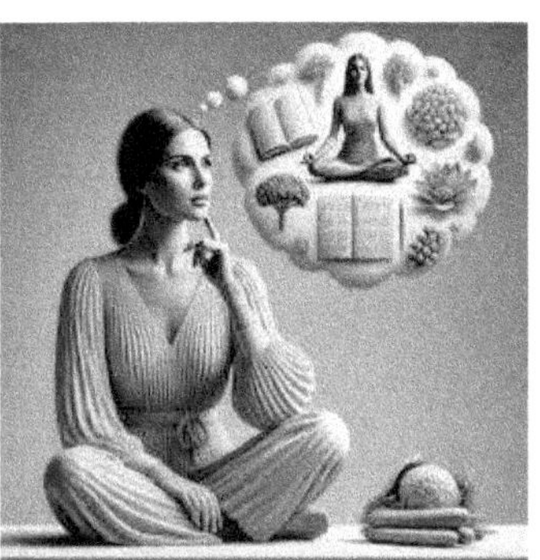

- What small changes can you make to your morning routine

- to support an anti-inflammatory lifestyle?

- How can you incorporate mindfulness practices into your daily schedule?

- What resources (books, podcasts, workshops) can you explore to enhance your understanding of anti-inflammatory living?

This reflection encourages mindfulness and intentionality, guiding you to identify opportunities for growth and integration in your daily life.

6.1 ADAPTING THE DIET FOR FAMILY AND FRIENDS

Picture your kitchen bustling with activity, the heart of your home where loved ones gather. Here, the aromas of a shared meal bring everyone together, regardless of dietary preferences. Inclusivity is vital in creating meals that satisfy diverse tastes and needs, primarily when you aim to maintain an anti-inflammatory lifestyle. One of the challenges is preparing meals that cater to both vegetarians and meat-eaters. A versatile dish like a hearty vegetable stir-fry can bridge this gap. Offer a base of colorful veggies and tofu for those who prefer plant-based options while providing a side of grilled chicken or shrimp for others. This approach ensures everyone enjoys the same meal, fostering a sense of unity. Similarly, offering gluten-free or nut-free options is essential when accommodating allergies or sensitivities. Use gluten-free pasta or rice noodles and substitute nut-based ingredients with seeds or legumes to maintain flavor and nutrition.

Planning family meals can be both an art and a science, requiring consideration of everyone's likes and dislikes while adhering to anti-inflammatory principles. Creating a weekly family meal plan can streamline this process. Begin by gathering input from each family member, encouraging them to suggest dishes they enjoy. This collaboration ensures variety and makes everyone feel involved in the decision-making. Once you've collected ideas, rotate your favorite meals to keep things interesting and prevent monotony. This approach allows you to balance familiarity with new culinary experiences, making meal times enjoyable and engaging. Planning meals together creates a sense of anticipation and excitement, turning dinner into a shared experience rather than a chore.

Involving family members in cooking is a beautiful way to deepen connections and share the responsibility of meal preparation. Assign tasks based on skill levels, allowing everyone to contribute in a meaningful way. Younger children might enjoy washing vegetables or setting the table, while older kids can do more complex tasks like chopping or seasoning. Hosting family cooking nights can be a delightful tradition where everyone gathers to try new recipes together. These evenings are opportunities for laughter, learning, and bonding as you explore different cuisines and flavors. They also instill valuable cooking skills and a love for wholesome food, laying the foundation for healthy habits.

For families with picky eaters, introducing new foods can be a challenge. Strategies that focus on gradual exposure and creativity can make a difference. Start by introducing new foods gradually, pairing them with familiar flavors to ease the transition. For instance, add a handful of spinach to a favorite pasta dish or blend some berries into a beloved smoothie. This approach allows picky eaters to explore new tastes without feeling overwhelmed. Fun presentation techniques like food art can entice hesitant eaters to try something new. Arranging veggies in colorful patterns or using cookie cutters to create fun shapes can make meals more appealing, turning dinner into a playful experience.

Ultimately, adapting to an anti-inflammatory diet for family and friends is about creating meals that celebrate diversity and inclusivity. It's about finding joy in cooking and eating together, where every dish tells a story, and every meal is an opportunity to connect. By embracing this approach, you nurture both your body and your relationships, fostering an environment of health and happiness.

6.2 NAVIGATING HOLIDAYS AND SPECIAL OCCASIONS

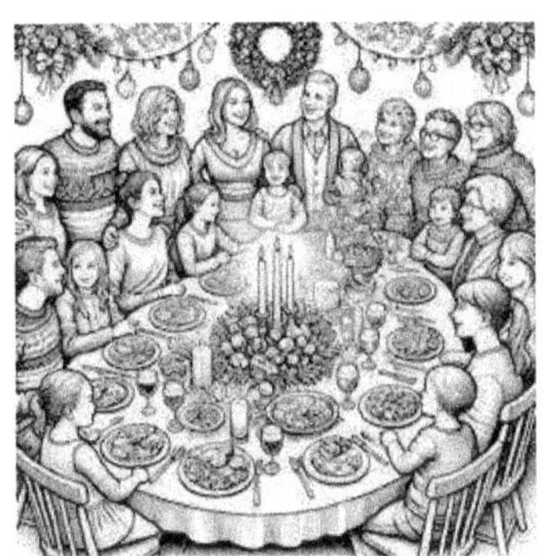

Holidays and special occasions often bring a sense of joy and celebration, yet they can also present unique challenges when maintaining an anti-inflammatory lifestyle. Amidst the festive atmosphere, buffet-style gatherings can become a minefield of temptation. The sight of rich and indulgent foods, enticingly displayed, can make it challenging to adhere to health goals. The key to navigating these events lies in balancing indulgence with mindful eating. Before attending a gathering, consider having a light, nutritious snack to curb your hunger and prevent overeating. This simple step ensures you approach the buffet with a clear mind, allowing you to make thoughtful choices rather than succumbing to impulse. When you fill your plate, focus on colorful vegetables, lean proteins, and whole grains, which satisfy and align with your dietary objectives.

Hosting or attending events can also be an opportunity to uphold your anti-inflammatory goals while sharing them with others. One effective strategy is to bring a healthy dish to share, ensuring at least one option fits within your dietary framework. A vibrant roasted vegetable platter with herb-infused dips can be a visually appealing centerpiece and a delicious, healthful choice. Infused water stations featuring an array of fruits and herbs, like mint and citrus slices, offer a refreshing alternative to sugary beverages. When attending events, communicate your dietary needs to hosts in advance. A simple conversation can open the door to understanding and accommodating your preferences, making it easier for everyone to enjoy the celebration together.

Celebrations offer the perfect canvas for creativity in the kitchen, where festive recipes can shine without straying from an anti-inflammatory path. Imagine a table adorned with dishes that delight the palate and nourish the body. A quinoa salad enriched with pomegranate seeds, walnuts, and a lemon-tahini dressing can provide flavor and nutrients. For those with a sweet tooth, a dessert of baked apples with cinnamon and a touch of maple syrup offers a comforting yet wholesome treat. These recipes fit the occasion and demonstrate that healthful eating need not sacrifice taste or enjoyment.

Building new traditions that align with health goals can transform how you approach holidays and special occasions. Consider organizing active outings, such as a family hike or a walk in the park, which allow you to connect with loved ones while staying active. These activities foster a sense of togetherness and provide a healthy counterbalance to the indulgences that often accompany celebrations. Hosting cooking workshops for friends and family can also be a rewarding endeavor. Gather together in the kitchen to explore new recipes, each contributing to a dish that aligns with an anti-inflammatory lifestyle. This shared experience enhances culinary skills and deepens connections, creating lasting memories beyond the event.

The key to successfully navigating holidays and special occasions is approaching them intentionally and creatively. You can enjoy these celebrations without compromising your health goals by preparing for challenges, engaging with others about your dietary needs, and building new, health-focused traditions. It's about finding joy in the process, discovering new flavors, and creating lasting memories with those you cherish.

6.3 SUSTAINING LONG-TERM HEALTH BENEFITS

Imagine setting the foundation for a healthier future, where every choice you make today contributes to your well-being tomorrow. Establishing lifelong habits is the cornerstone of sustaining the benefits of an anti-inflammatory lifestyle. Regular exercise is not just about building muscle or losing weight; it's about maintaining vitality and preventing inflammation. Committing to a consistent exercise routine improves circulation, strengthens the heart, and supports joint health. Whether it's a brisk walk in the park, a yoga class, or lifting weights, the key is to find activities you enjoy and can do regularly. These moments of movement become integral parts of your life, reinforcing your commitment to health. Alongside physical activity, prioritizing mental health is vital. Stress management techniques like meditation, deep breathing, and creative pursuits like painting or writing can significantly reduce stress-induced inflammation. These practices provide the mental space needed to navigate life's challenges with resilience and calm, ensuring that your health journey is comprehensive and balanced.

Regular health assessments serve as a compass, guiding you on your path to well-being. You can make proactive decisions tailored to your body's needs by staying informed about your health metrics. Annual check-ups with your healthcare provider offer an opportunity to monitor essential health markers, from blood pressure to cholesterol levels, providing a snapshot of your overall health. Keeping a record of these assessments allows you to track changes and trends, helping you identify areas requiring attention. In addition to general health checks, monitoring inflammation markers such as C-reactive protein

(CRP) can offer insights into your body's inflammatory state. This information can be invaluable in assessing the effectiveness of your lifestyle choices and making necessary adjustments. By taking control of your health data, you empower yourself to make informed decisions that support long-term vitality.

Flexibility and adaptability are vital components of any successful health strategy. Life is dynamic, with changes and challenges that can impact your well-being. Embracing flexibility means understanding that your needs may evolve over time. Adjusting dietary choices to accommodate life changes, whether due to aging, lifestyle shifts, or new health information, is crucial. This adaptability ensures that your approach remains relevant and practical, allowing you to respond to your body's evolving requirements. Staying open to new research and techniques is equally important. The field of nutrition and wellness is ever-changing, with emerging studies offering fresh perspectives on health management. By remaining curious and engaged, you can incorporate new insights that enhance your lifestyle, ensuring that your commitment to health is both innovative and informed.

Sharing success stories of individuals who have reaped long-term benefits from an anti- inflammatory lifestyle can be incredibly motivating. Consider the family who transformed their health by embracing whole foods and regular physical activity. Their journey wasn't without challenges, but the rewards—improved energy, reduced inflammation, and a stronger sense of connection —made every effort worthwhile. Testimonials from older adults experiencing renewed vitality and energy offer further inspiration. These individuals have witnessed firsthand the power of sustained health practices, from improved mobility to enhanced cognitive function. Their stories remind us that it's never too late to adopt positive changes and that the benefits of an anti-inflammatory lifestyle can extend well into later life. These real-life examples highlight the profound impact of commitment and perseverance, encouraging us to envision a future where health is a lifelong priority.

In conclusion, sustaining long-term health benefits involves cultivating habits that support your body and mind, monitoring your progress with regular assessments, and embracing flexibility in your approach. As you integrate these principles into your life, you lay the foundation for a healthier, more vibrant future. This chapter serves as a reminder that health is a continuous journey that evolves with each choice you make. The next chapter will delve into practical meal planning and recipes, providing tools to support your anti-inflammatory lifestyle further.

CHAPTER 7

ADDRESSING COMMON PAIN POINTS

Imagine standing in your kitchen, the clock ticking towards late afternoon. You've had a long day, and the allure of a quick snack is calling your name. The craving isn't just for food; it's a beckoning comfort, a momentary escape from stress or boredom. Such cravings often arise not from hunger but from emotions and environmental cues that entangle our eating habits in a web of complexity. Stress and emotions are powerful triggers, leading many to reach for food as solace. Food can seem like a friend in moments of anxiety or sadness, offering a temporary balm to emotional wounds. Social settings, too, often encourage indulgence, where the sights and smells of shared meals act as subtle invitations to indulge beyond our intentions.

Recognizing these triggers is the first step in managing cravings. It's essential to understand that emotional eating often stems from a deeper need for comfort or distraction from unpleasant emotions. This type of hunger appears suddenly, demanding specific comfort foods and leading to mindless consumption, often accompanied by guilt afterward. Social gatherings can also amplify cravings. Surrounded by friends and laughter, the pressure to partake can be overwhelming, sometimes resulting in choices that don't align with your health goals. By identifying these patterns, you can start unraveling their hold on your eating habits.

To combat cravings effectively, consider shifting your focus toward actionable strategies that empower you to regain control. Begin by drinking a glass of water before meals. This simple act can help curb appetite by promoting a sense of fullness, reducing the likelihood of overeating.

Practicing mindful eating further enhances awareness, encouraging you to savor each bite and recognize when you are genuinely satiated. By paying attention to the sensations of eating, you can differentiate between physical hunger and emotional need, fostering a healthier relationship with food.

Healthy substitutions offer another avenue for satisfying cravings without derailing your diet. Instead of reaching for a bag of chips, consider roasted chickpeas. They provide a satisfying crunch and are rich in fiber and protein, helping you feel full longer. For those with a sweet tooth, choose fruit and yogurt over ice cream. A bowl of mixed berries with a dollop of Greek yogurt can satisfy sugar cravings while delivering antioxidants and probiotics that support your health. These substitutions not only fulfill cravings but also align with your anti-inflammatory goals.

Building new habits is crucial in transforming your relationship with food. Establishing regular meal times prevents grazing, helping to stabilize blood sugar levels and reduce impulsive snacking. Planning your meals and snacks throughout the day creates a structured routine supporting balanced eating. Incorporating a variety of flavors and textures into your meals can also prevent monotony, making it easier to stick to healthy choices. Experiment with herbs, spices, and diverse ingredients to keep meals exciting and satisfying, reducing the temptation to stray to less healthy options.

7.1 CRAVING REFLECTION EXERCISE

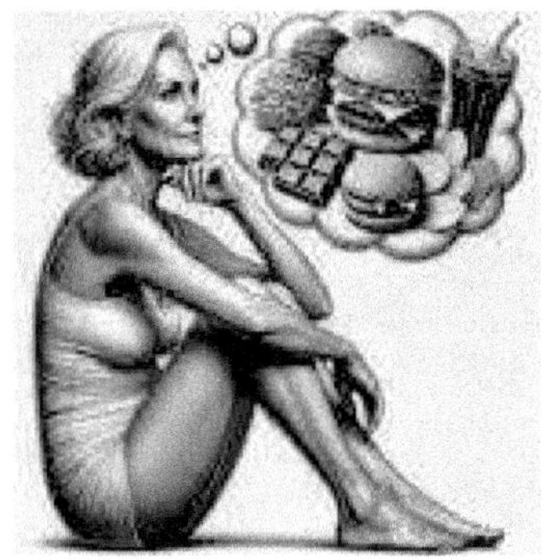

Set aside a few moments each day to jot down when and what you crave and any emotions or situations that might have triggered the craving. Over time, this exercise can help you identify patterns and better understand your triggers.

As you embark on this journey to manage cravings, remember that it's about progress, not perfection. Each step, identifying a trigger, substituting a healthier option, or forming a new habit, is a step toward a more balanced and fulfilling way of eating. Cravings need not control you; with awareness and intention, you can master them, paving the way for a healthier, more mindful life.

7.2 EATING OUT WITHOUT COMPROMISING YOUR DIET

Dining out can be a delightful and daunting experience, especially when you're committed to maintaining an anti-inflammatory diet. The challenge often lies in navigating menus that are often laden with enticing but only sometimes healthful options. However, with some knowledge and forethought, you can make choices that align with your dietary goals. One effective strategy is to ask for dressings and sauces on the side, allowing you to control the amount you consume and preventing excess calories and added sugars that can contribute to inflammation. Similarly, opting for grilled or baked options instead of fried can significantly reduce unhealthy fats. Grilled chicken or baked fish are delicious and align with anti-inflammatory principles, offering a healthier alternative without sacrificing taste.

Communication with restaurant staff can also play a pivotal role in maintaining your diet when eating out. Feel free to request whole grains instead of refined ones. Many restaurants are happy to accommodate dietary needs, offering brown rice or wholegrain bread instead of their processed counterparts. Additionally, inquire about ingredient substitutions. A dish prepared with heavy cream might be made with a lighter broth or coconut milk upon request. These adjustments can transform a meal, keeping it flavorful while aligning with your health objectives. Being transparent and polite about your dietary preferences ensures that your needs are met without feeling like an imposition.

Social dynamics in dining settings can sometimes pose challenges, with peer pressure nudging you towards choices that might not fit your dietary commitments. To navigate these situations, consider selecting restaurants with diverse menus offering various options. This way, everyone can find something they enjoy, and you won't feel restricted. Being assertive about your dietary boundaries is crucial. Politely but firmly express your preferences, setting an example and potentially inspiring others to consider healthier options. It's important to remember that maintaining your health is a priority, and those who care about you will respect your choices.

Planning ahead can make dining out a stress-free experience. With the digital age at your fingertips, researching menus online before you go can provide clarity and confidence. Many restaurants list their menus on their websites, allowing you to identify dishes that align with your diet in advance. Take note of eateries known for offering healthy options, such as those that emphasize fresh, local ingredients or have a reputation for accommodating special dietary needs. Choosing these establishments not only supports your lifestyle but also reduces the anxiety of making hasty decisions when faced with a menu of tempting options.

Informed choices, effective communication, and a proactive approach are key to enjoying meals out without compromising your diet. This balance allows you to savor the social and culinary aspects of dining out while maintaining your commitment to health.

7.3 BUDGET-FRIENDLY ANTI-INFLAMMATORY CHOICES

Focusing on cost-effective ingredients can make a significant difference when you want to maintain an anti-inflammatory diet without breaking the bank. One of the simplest ways to save money while still eating healthy is to purchase in-season fruits and vegetables. Not only are these produce items at their peak flavor and nutrition, but they're also more affordable due to their abundance. Think of juicy tomatoes in the summer or crisp apples in the fall. These seasonal gems can significantly reduce your grocery bill while ensuring your meals are bursting with flavor and nutrients. Another economic powerhouse is beans and lentils. These legumes are not only rich in protein and fiber but also versatile enough to be included in a variety of dishes. Whether making a hearty chili or a refreshing salad, beans, and lentils provide the protein punch needed to keep you satiated and keep your inflammation in check.

Innovative shopping techniques can further stretch your budget while maintaining a healthy diet. Buying in bulk is a practical approach, allowing you to stock up on staples like grains, nuts, and seeds at a reduced price per unit. Once home, dividing these items into portions ensures they remain fresh over time and are easy to grab when needed. Comparing prices at local markets and supermarkets can also lead to savings. Often, local markets offer competitive pricing on fresh produce and bulk items, allowing you to find the best deals without compromising on quality. By being strategic with where and how you shop, you can enjoy the benefits of an anti- inflammatory diet without financial stress.

Meal planning is another effective strategy for managing food costs and minimizing waste. By creating a shopping list based on weekly menus, you can avoid impulse buys and ensure you purchase only what you need. This approach helps you stick to your budget and reduces the likelihood of food waste. Using leftovers creatively can transform yesterday's dinner into today's lunch, stretching your meals further. For example, leftover roasted vegetables can be repurposed into a frittata or added to a soup, maximizing their use and reducing waste. Meal planning encourages thoughtful consumption, fostering an environment where every ingredient is valued and utilized.

Including budget-friendly recipes in your repertoire is key to sustaining an anti-inflammatory lifestyle. Consider hearty vegetable soups that combine inexpensive produce like carrots, potatoes, and onions. These soups are both warming and nutritious and incredibly cost- effective, allowing you to make large batches that can be enjoyed over several days. Similarly, stir-fry dishes with budget-friendly frozen vegetables offer a quick and nutritious meal option. Frozen vegetables are often picked at peak ripeness and flash-frozen to preserve their nutrients, making them a convenient and healthy choice. Using these ingredients as the base for your meals, you can create flavorful, anti-inflammatory dishes that nourish your body without straining your wallet.

7.4 OVERCOMING WEIGHT MANAGEMENT CHALLENGES

In the intricate web of health, inflammation often plays a subtle yet powerful role in weight gain. It's not just about the number on the scale; it's about understanding how your body processes and stores energy. Chronic inflammation can disrupt this balance, affecting metabolism and making weight management more challenging. One of the critical pathways involves insulin resistance, a condition where your cells become less responsive to insulin, the hormone that helps regulate blood sugar levels. When insulin resistance develops, your body struggles to manage glucose effectively, often leading to increased fat storage and weight gain. This cycle can be exacerbated by inflammation, as the body's persistent state of alert can further impair metabolic processes. Recognizing this connection is vital for addressing weight issues holistically, focusing not just on calories but on the underlying factors that influence weight.

A gradual approach is often the most effective way to achieve sustainable weight loss. Begin with portion control, a practice that emphasizes quality over quantity. Paying attention to portion sizes allows you to enjoy the foods you love without overindulging. This doesn't mean deprivation; it means savoring each bite and understanding your body's hunger signals.

Balanced meals are also vital, ensuring each plate mixes protein, healthy fats, and complex carbohydrates. This balance helps maintain energy levels and keeps you satisfied longer, reducing the temptation to reach for unhealthy snacks. Alongside dietary adjustments, increasing physical activity is crucial. Find exercises you enjoy, whether dancing, hiking, or cycling. The goal is to move more naturally and joyfully rather than a chore.

A positive body image and mindset can transform your journey toward better health. Rather than fixating on numbers, focus on wellness. Celebrate non-scale victories, like increased energy, improved mood, or the ability to move more freely. These moments are powerful reminders of progress that goes beyond physical appearance. Practicing self-compassion is equally important. Treat yourself with kindness and patience, recognizing that setbacks are part of the process. Mindfulness can help here, offering a way to connect with your body and its needs without judgment. By fostering a mindset that values wellness over weight, you create a supportive environment for lasting change.

Personalized solutions are fundamental to effective weight management. Each person's journey is unique, shaped by individual circumstances and health needs. Set realistic goals that reflect where you are now, not where you think you should be. This might mean aiming for a specific fitness milestone or improving a health marker rather than a particular weight. Consulting with healthcare professionals can provide tailored advice and support, ensuring your plans align with your health requirements. They can help you navigate challenges, offering insights and adjustments as needed. This personalized approach ensures that your weight management efforts are effective and sustainable.

Remember that weight management is a multifaceted process. You can achieve a healthier balance by addressing inflammation, embracing gradual changes, and maintaining a positive mindset. This chapter has explored how inflammation influences weight and offered strategies for overcoming related challenges. The next chapter will delve into more specific recipes and meal plans to support your anti-inflammatory lifestyle, helping you put these principles into practice.

CHAPTER 8

RECIPES AND CULINARY
INSPIRATION

Picture your kitchen as a vibrant painting, each ingredient a bold brushstroke adding depth and character to your culinary canvas. The rich reds of tomatoes, the verdant greens of kale, and the earthy browns of mushrooms combine to create a meal and an experience. As you stand at the counter, you hold the power to transform these raw elements into a nourishing masterpiece. Embracing vegetarian and vegan dishes is not merely about removing animal products but celebrating plant-based foods' diverse flavors and nutrients. These meals are kind to your body and the planet, contributing to a more sustainable and health-conscious lifestyle.

Opting for plant-based eating significantly reduces inflammation and adds variety to your diet. It emphasizes nutrient density and fiber content, crucial in maintaining health. Vegetables, fruits, grains, and legumes provide essential vitamins and minerals, supporting bodily functions and reducing chronic inflammation. Fiber, abundant in plant foods, aids digestion and stabilizes blood sugar levels, creating a balanced internal environment.

Beyond personal health, plant- based diets offer environmental benefits. They require fewer natural resources and produce less greenhouse gas emissions than diets high in animal products. This shift toward sustainable eating supports individual well-being and the planet, creating a harmonious balance between people and nature.

Incorporating versatile plant proteins into your meals is key to ensuring adequate nutrition. Lentils and chickpeas are excellent sources of protein, perfect for hearty stews that warm the soul and satisfy hunger. These legumes provide essential amino acids, making them a staple in vegetarian and vegan kitchens. Tofu and tempeh, derived from soybeans, offer another avenue for plant-based protein. Their mild flavors make them ideal for stir-fries, absorbing seasonings and sauces beautifully. By experimenting with these proteins, you can create delicious and nutritious meals that meet your dietary needs without relying on animal products. These ingredients provide the building blocks for a balanced diet and invite creativity and exploration in the kitchen.

For those looking to craft complete meals, consider a quinoa and black bean salad with lime vinaigrette. This dish combines the nutty flavor of quinoa with the hearty texture of black beans, offering a satisfying and nutrient-rich meal. The lime vinaigrette adds a refreshing tang, elevating the dish with a burst of citrus.

Alternatively, a roasted vegetable medley with tahini dressing highlights the natural sweetness of seasonal produce, complemented by tahini's creamy, nutty flavor. These recipes showcase the potential of plant-based ingredients to create balanced, satisfying meals that support health and well-being. They demonstrate that vegetarian and vegan dishes can be rich in flavor, texture, and nutrition, offering a feast for the palate and the body.

Creativity in the kitchen encourages you to experiment with ingredients and cooking methods. Grilled portobello mushrooms make excellent burger alternatives, offering a meaty texture and smoky flavor that can satisfy even the most devout carnivore. Pair them with a whole-grain bun and your favorite toppings for a satisfying meal that respects your health goals and taste buds.

Alternatively, spiralized zucchini noodles with avocado pesto provide a fresh take on a classic dish, combining the lightness of zucchini with the creamy richness of avocado. This dish is delicious and visually appealing, transforming simple ingredients into a gourmet experience. By embracing creativity, you open the door to endless possibilities in plant-based cooking, discovering new flavors and combinations that delight the senses and nourish the body.

8.1 PLANT-BASED COOKING CHALLENGE

Set a goal to create three new plant-based meals this week. Use this checklist to guide your exploration:

- Choose a base: Quinoa, lentils, or chickpeas
- Select a protein: Tofu, tempeh, or beans
- Add vegetables: Kale, bell peppers, or mushrooms
- Experiment with flavors: Lime, tahini, or avocado
- Document your creations with photos and notes on flavors and textures.

This challenge encourages you to explore the vast world of plant-based cooking and inspires you to incorporate more vegetarian and vegan dishes into your routine. This step will enhance your culinary skills and support your journey toward a healthier, more sustainable lifestyle.

8.2 GLUTEN-FREE AND DAIRY-FREE RECIPES

For many, going gluten-free or dairy-free isn't just a dietary preference; it's a necessity driven by health concerns. Gluten, a protein found in wheat, barley, and rye, can trigger inflammation in susceptible individuals, potentially exacerbating conditions like celiac disease and non-celiac gluten sensitivity.

Similarly, dairy, mainly lactose and casein, can pose digestive challenges for those who are intolerant or allergic, leading to discomfort and inflammation. These sensitivities highlight the importance of creating recipes catering to specific dietary restrictions and supporting an anti-inflammatory lifestyle. Removing gluten and dairy alleviates potential triggers, and embracing options contributes to holistic well-being.

When it comes to crafting gluten-free and dairy-free dishes, the challenge lies in maintaining flavor and texture. Fortunately, a variety of alternative ingredients rise to the occasion. Almond flour, with its slightly nutty taste, is a fantastic substitute for wheat flour in baked goods, providing moisture and richness without the gluten. Coconut milk, known for its creamy texture and subtle sweetness, replaces dairy seamlessly in sweet and savory dishes. These alternatives allow you to enjoy your favorite meals without sacrificing taste or quality. With its cheesy flavor, nutritional yeast steps in as a dairy-free hero, perfect for sprinkling over pasta or incorporating into sauces for a hint of umami. These ingredients are the building blocks for delicious meals that nourish the body while respecting dictary needs.

Consider a baked sweet potato with chickpea curry, a satisfying dish that combines the earthiness of sweet potatoes with the warm spices of a chickpea curry. The sweet potatoes, roasted to perfection, serve as a comforting base, while the curry, rich in flavor and nutrients, offers protein and fiber. This meal is both gluten- and dairy-free and simple to prepare, fitting seamlessly into daily life. Another favorite is the cauliflower crust pizza, topped with a fresh tomato sauce. This pizza captures the essence of a traditional pie while replacing gluten-laden crusts with one made from cauliflower. The result is a dish that delivers all the satisfaction of pizza without inflammatory ingredients. These recipes highlight how gluten- and dairy-free options can be practical and delicious, providing sustenance and joy.

Adapting traditional recipes to fit gluten-free and dairy-free parameters requires a few strategic adjustments. Arrowroot powder emerges as a reliable ally for thickening sauces and soups, offering a gluten-free alternative to conventional thickeners like flour. It blends smoothly without altering flavor, ensuring your dishes maintain their intended taste and consistency. With its rich buttery texture, coconut oil becomes a go-to substitute for butter in baking and cooking. Its subtle sweetness complements savory and sweet dishes, adding depth and richness. By making these adjustments, you can transform beloved recipes into versions that align with your dietary needs, ensuring you never compromise on flavor or enjoyment.

Navigating the world of gluten-free and dairy-free cooking opens up a realm of possibilities, encouraging creativity and experimentation. Each recipe allows you to explore new flavors and textures, expanding your culinary repertoire while supporting your health goals. This approach fosters a sense of empowerment, enabling you to take control of your diet and make choices that align with your body's needs. You create meals that taste great and promote an anti- inflammatory lifestyle by embracing alternative ingredients and techniques.

8.3 INCORPORATING ANTI-INFLAMMATORY SPICES

Imagine opening your spice cabinet to vibrant colors and intoxicating aromas. Each jar holds the promise of vibrant flavors and healing potential. Spices have been used for centuries, not just to enhance the taste of food but to promote health. Certain spices stand out for their powerful properties in reducing inflammation. Take turmeric, for example. Its active ingredient, curcumin, is known for its potent anti-inflammatory effects. This golden spice can transform a simple dish into a healthful powerhouse, working to soothe inflammation in the body. Similarly, capsaicin, found in chili peppers, not only adds a fiery kick to your meals but also supports the reduction of inflammation. Capsaicin works by inhibiting specific pathways that lead to inflammatory responses, making it a tasty ally in your dietary arsenal.

Beyond these, other spices offer both a culinary delight and health benefits. With its warm and slightly spicy flavor, ginger is celebrated for its digestive benefits. It aids digestion and reduces nausea, making it a versatile addition to sweet and savory dishes. Whether brewing it in a tea or grating it into a marinade, ginger can ease digestive discomfort and support a healthy gut.

Cinnamon, another staple in many kitchens, plays a crucial role in regulating blood sugar levels. Its sweet and woody aroma can elevate any dish, while its health benefits work quietly in the background, helping to maintain stable blood sugar and reduce the risk of diabetes. Incorporating these spices into your meals enhances flavor and helps your body fight inflammation.

To fully experience these spices' benefits, consider incorporating them into your cooking through flavorful recipes. A turmeric and ginger rice pilaf combines the earthy tones of turmeric with the zesty warmth of ginger, creating a comforting and nourishing dish. The rice, infused with these spices, becomes a fragrant base for any meal, perfect for pairing with proteins or vegetables. For a snack with a kick, try spicy roasted chickpeas with paprika. These crunchy treats offer a satisfying bite, with paprika and capsaicin working together to provide flavor and anti-inflammatory benefits. These recipes highlight how incorporating spices can transform everyday meals into healthful creations, showcasing their potential to improve taste and wellness.

Encouraging creativity with spice blends allows you to tailor flavors to your personal preferences, creating unique dishes that reflect your culinary style. Homemade curry powder, for instance, can be adjusted to suit your taste, whether you prefer it mild or with a bit of heat. Combining turmeric, cumin, coriander, and a pinch of chili powder creates a blend perfect for seasoning everything from vegetables to meats. Similarly, crafting your own herb and spice blends for seasoning provides endless possibilities. Mix oregano, thyme, and rosemary with garlic powder for a Mediterranean twist, or combine ginger, cinnamon, and cloves for a warming, aromatic blend. These blends personalize your cooking and ensure you receive the maximum health benefits from these powerful spices.

8.4 INTERNATIONAL CUISINE WITH AN ANTI-INFLAMMATORY TWIST

Imagine your kitchen transforming into a global culinary playground, where each dish tells a story of tradition and innovation. By exploring global flavors, you can infuse your meals with the rich tapestries of Mediterranean, Middle Eastern, and Asian influences while embracing an anti- inflammatory lifestyle. These cuisines naturally lend themselves to healthful eating, emphasizing fresh herbs and spices that elevate simple ingredients. Whether it's the aromatic basil and oregano in a Mediterranean dish or the fragrant cumin and coriander in Middle Eastern fare, these flavors tantalize your taste buds and support your body's well-being.

Adapting traditional recipes to fit an anti-inflammatory diet involves preserving authenticity while reducing ingredients that may contribute to inflammation. Take, for instance, the beloved Thai green curry. By substituting coconut milk for dairy, you retain the creamy richness of the dish while ensuring it aligns with anti-inflammatory principles. Full of vibrant vegetables, this version offers a variety of flavors without the need for inflammatory additives. Similarly, a Moroccan tagine can be reimagined with chickpeas and apricots, creating a hearty, plant-based meal that sings with the warmth of cinnamon and ginger. These adaptations demonstrate that you don't have to sacrifice tradition for health; you can harmonize the two to enjoy the best of both worlds.

For those who love to experiment, fusion recipes present an exciting opportunity to blend different culinary traditions, resulting in unique flavors that surprise and delight. Imagine creating quinoa sushi rolls, where the nutty grains replace traditional rice and creamy avocado with a sprinkling of sesame seeds for added texture and flavor. These rolls offer a nutrient-packed alternative to conventional sushi, delivering both taste and health benefits. Or consider Indian- inspired lentil tacos, where lentils, rich in protein and fiber, are spiced with cumin and coriander and then topped with a zesty cilantro chutney. These tacos bring together the heartiness of Indian cuisine and the boldness of Mexican flavors, creating a dish as nourishing as delicious.

The nutritional benefits of incorporating global ingredients into your diet are profound. Olive oil, a staple in Mediterranean cooking, is revered for its heart-healthy monounsaturated fats and antioxidants, which help reduce inflammation and protect against chronic diseases. Drizzling it over salads or using it as a base for sautéing vegetables can enhance flavor and health.

Meanwhile, fermented foods like kimchi, common in Asian cuisine, are rich in probiotics that support gut health and reduce inflammation. Including a side of kimchi with your meal can add a spicy kick while promoting a balanced digestive system. By embracing these diverse ingredients, you diversify your palate and bolster your body's defenses against inflammation.

In exploring international cuisine, you're invited to embrace creativity and curiosity. Whether it's trying a new spice blend or reinventing a classic dish, the possibilities are endless. Each recipe becomes a canvas where flavors, textures, and colors combine to create something extraordinary. This chapter has guided you through the vibrant world of global culinary traditions, showing how they can be adapted to an anti-inflammatory lifestyle without compromising taste or authenticity. As you experiment with these recipes, remember that food is not just sustenance; it expresses culture, history, and health. Integrating these elements into your meals enriches your dining experience and supports your journey toward a healthier, more balanced life.

With these flavorful inspirations in mind, you are now ready to explore the practical elements of planning and preparing meals that fit your busy lifestyle, ensuring that nourishment and convenience go hand in hand.

CHAPTER 9

PRACTICAL MEAL PLANNING

Imagine walking into your kitchen, where the promise of a week filled with delicious, healthful meals awaits. Yet, the chaos of everyday life often turns meal planning into a daunting task. Between work deadlines, family commitments, and social events, finding time to prepare balanced meals can feel like trying to fit a puzzle piece into a mismatched board. But what if this process could be simplified, turning mealtime into a stress-free, nourishing experience? In this chapter, we'll explore practical meal-planning strategies that cater to busy adults, ensuring you can enjoy the health benefits of an anti-inflammatory diet without the hassle.

9.1 MEAL PLANNING FOR BUSY ADULTS

Time-saving techniques are the cornerstone of effective meal planning. Imagine the luxury of fresh groceries arriving at your doorstep. Utilizing grocery delivery services can save significant time, allowing you to focus on meal preparation rather than the logistics of shopping. Many services offer customizable lists, enabling you to select anti-inflammatory staples such as leafy greens, whole grains, and lean proteins. This convenience allows you to plan your meals precisely, ensuring you have all the necessary ingredients without the stress of last-minute store runs.

Setting aside a specific day for meal prep can transform your weekly routine. Choose a day that suits your schedule: a Sunday afternoon or a quiet weekday evening. Dedicate this time to preparing meals in advance, turning it into a ritual that signals the start of a week filled with nutritious eating. Create a weekly menu outlining breakfast, lunch, dinner, and snacks. This proactive approach organizes your week and helps you maintain a balanced diet. Once your menu is set, start prepping ingredients. Chop vegetables, marinate proteins, and portion out snacks. Doing this minimizes daily cooking time, making sticking to your dietary goals easier.

Versatile recipes are your best ally in meal planning. Imagine roasting a tray of vegetables that can be transformed throughout the week. On Monday, they might accompany grilled chicken seasoned with herbs and spices to create a savory dinner. By Wednesday, those same vegetables could be repurposed into a hearty salad or tossed with whole-grain pasta for a satisfying lunch. Proteins like grilled chicken or tofu are equally adaptable, serving as the centerpiece for various dishes. These versatile ingredients allow you to maintain culinary excitement, ensuring each meal feels fresh and new despite reusing core components.

Nutritional balance is crucial when planning meals. Each dish should offer a well-rounded profile of macronutrients, providing the energy and nutrients your body needs. Aim to balance proteins, carbohydrates, and fats, ensuring that each meal delivers sustained energy and satiety.

Incorporate various colors and textures, not only for visual appeal but also to maximize nutritional diversity. A colorful plate often indicates a diverse range of nutrients, supporting everything from immune function to heart health. By focusing on balance, you create meals that are nourishing and delicious.

Weekly Meal Planning Chart

- Create a weekly meal planning chart that includes: Days of the week with slots for breakfast, lunch, dinner, and snacks
- A section for grocery lists to ensure all necessary ingredients are on hand
- Columns to track macronutrients and ensure balanced meals

This chart acts as a visual aid, guiding your meal preparation and helping you maintain a balanced, anti-inflammatory diet.

9.2 BATCH COOKING AND FREEZING ANTI-INFLAMMATORY MEALS

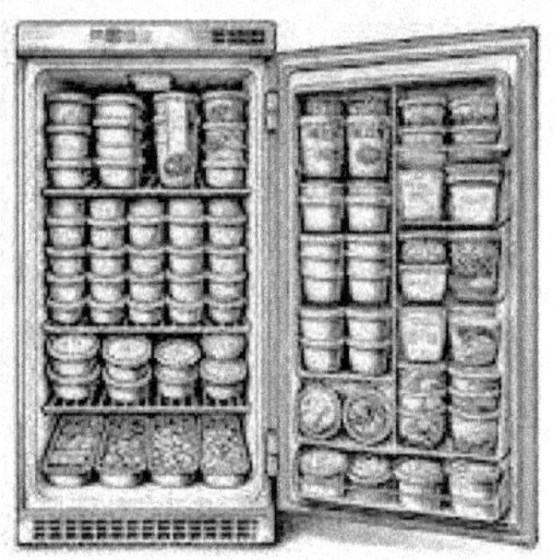

Batch cooking is a lifeline for those seeking to maintain a healthy diet amidst a whirlwind of responsibilities. By dedicating a few hours to preparing meals in large quantities, you can alleviate daily cooking stress and ensure you always have nourishing options on hand.

Imagine the relief of opening your freezer to find a variety of home-cooked meals ready to reheat.

Preparing soups and stews in bulk is particularly advantageous. Consider a rich vegetable stew simmering with herbs and spices that fill your kitchen with warmth and aroma. Once cooked, these meals can be portioned and frozen, ready to provide comfort and sustenance whenever needed.

Freezing meals effectively requires a few key techniques to maintain flavor and nutrition. Start by using airtight containers or freezer bags to prevent freezer burn, which can compromise taste and texture. Ensure minimal air is left in the packaging, which helps preserve the food's quality. Label each container or bag with the meal's name and the date it was prepared. This simple step prevents the dreaded freezer mystery meals and helps you track what needs to be eaten first. As you organize your freezer, consider grouping similar meals together for easy access, finding exactly what you're craving.

Some recipes naturally lend themselves to freezing, retaining their anti-inflammatory benefits even after being stored. Take, for instance, a hearty lentil and vegetable curry. Lentils are rich in protein and fiber, while vegetables provide essential vitamins and minerals. Spices like turmeric and cumin add depth of flavor and enhance the meal's anti-inflammatory properties. Another excellent option is quinoa and black bean chili. Quinoa offers a complete protein source, while black beans contain antioxidants. Together, they create a satisfying dish that freezes beautifully, ready to be enjoyed on any busy day.

Reheating frozen meals to their former glory requires a bit of finesse. For best results, thaw your chosen meal overnight in the refrigerator. This gentle thawing process helps maintain the dish's texture and flavor. When it's time to reheat, opt for the stovetop or microwave. If using the stovetop, heat the meal slowly over low to medium heat, stirring occasionally to ensure even warming. Cover the dish with a microwave-safe lid or wrap for microwave reheating, and heat in short intervals, stirring in between. This method prevents overcooking and helps retain moisture, giving you a meal that tastes as if it were freshly made.

9.3 QUICK AND EASY BREAKFASTS

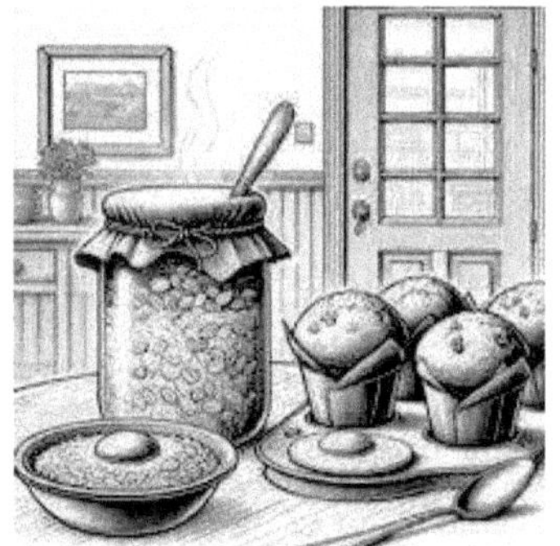

Picture the moment your morning begins. The sun peeks through the window, a gentle glow promising a fresh start. This is the perfect time to set a positive tone for the day with a nutritious breakfast. An anti-inflammatory breakfast acts as a foundation for both body and mind. It jumpstarts your metabolism, providing the energy needed to tackle the day's challenges. A balanced morning meal stabilizes blood sugar levels and enhances concentration, making those early hours more productive. Consider it the fuel that powers your daily endeavors, helping you stay focused and energized until lunchtime.

Imagine the simplicity of starting your day with overnight oats. The night before, mix rolled oats with chia seeds, your choice of milk, and a handful of berries. Let this mixture sit in the fridge, where it will transform into a creamy, satisfying breakfast ready to grab and go. The oats provide slow-releasing carbohydrates that keep hunger at bay, while chia seeds boost omega- 3s and fiber. Berries introduce flavor and antioxidants, making this meal delicious and nutritious. Alternatively, consider a smoothie with spinach, banana, and almond milk. This green powerhouse blends in moments, offering a refreshing start with minimal prep. The banana's natural sweetness complements the spinach's subtle earthiness, creating a harmonious balance that satisfies without overwhelming.

For those who prefer make-ahead options, egg muffins offer a savory solution. Whisk eggs with various vegetables, such as bell peppers, spinach, or tomatoes, and pour the mixture into a muffin tin. Bake until set, and you'll have a batch of portable, protein-rich breakfasts ready for the week. These muffins are flexible, allowing you to experiment with different veggies and spices to suit your taste. Homemade granola bars are another excellent choice.

Combine oats, nuts, seeds, and a touch of honey, press the mixture into a pan and bake. These bars are perfect for a quick breakfast on busy mornings, providing a combination of carbohydrates, healthy fats, and protein to keep you satisfied.

However, mornings can present challenges. Time often slips away, leaving little room for preparing a nutritious breakfast. Combat this by preparing breakfast the night before. Set out ingredients or fully prepare meals to avoid the morning rush. For those with limited appetite, opt for light, easy-to-digest options. A small serving of yogurt with fruit or a simple smoothie can provide the necessary nutrients without feeling heavy. These solutions ensure that even the most hectic mornings start on the right foot, nourishing your body and setting a positive tone for the day ahead.

Breakfast dilemmas are common but need not derail your commitment to a healthy diet. Incorporate quick and easy solutions that align with your lifestyle, ensuring breakfast becomes a seamless part of your routine. By prioritizing a nutritious start, you support your physical health and create a mental framework that encourages daily mindful choices. Each morning presents an opportunity to nourish and energize, turning breakfast into a celebration of well-being.

9.4 FAMILY-FRIENDLY MEAL IDEAS

Picture the scene: a lively kitchen filled with the chatter of family members, each contributing to the meal in their own way. This is the essence of family-friendly dining—bringing everyone together over meals that satisfy diverse tastes while fostering a sense of community. To appeal to adults and children, meals must be versatile and engaging. Customizable taco nights are a great example. Lay out a spread of tortillas, seasoned proteins like chicken or beans, and a colorful array of toppings such as avocado, tomatoes, and shredded cheese. Let each family member build their own taco, making choices that suit their preferences. This approach caters to individual tastes and encourages creativity and participation, turning dinner into a collaborative event.

Another adaptable option is a build-your-own salad bar. Set up a variety of fresh vegetables, proteins like grilled chicken or chickpeas, and toppings such as nuts, seeds, and dressings. This setup empowers each person to craft a meal that aligns with their dietary needs and flavor preferences. For children, it becomes an opportunity to explore new ingredients in a fun and interactive way. Encourage them to try a few new items by incorporating a game element, like who can create the most colorful salad. This strategy makes meals more enjoyable and introduces kids to healthy eating habits, emphasizing variety and balance.

Incorporating fun and interactive elements into meal preparation can transform the cooking process into an enjoyable family activity. Consider hosting a pizza night with healthy toppings. Prepare whole-grain pizza dough and set out a selection of toppings— fresh vegetables, lean meats, and flavorful herbs. Allow each person to create their masterpiece, experimenting with different combinations. Baking the pizzas together adds anticipation and excitement, as everyone looks forward to tasting their creations.

Similarly, DIY sushi rolls can be a hit. Provide sheets of nori, sticky rice, and a range of fillings like cucumber, avocado, and smoked salmon. Rolling sushi becomes a shared experience, blending culinary skills with creativity.

While fun is important, balancing nutrition and flavor ensures that family meals are enjoyable and beneficial. Use herbs and spices to enhance flavor without relying on excess salt or sugar. Fresh basil, cilantro, and rosemary can elevate dishes, adding depth and interest. Balancing proteins, veggies, and grains in each meal supports a well-rounded diet. Aim for a mix of textures and colors, creating visually appealing plates that entice even the pickiest eaters. This balance satisfies taste buds and delivers essential nutrients, supporting health for all family members.

Addressing picky eaters can be a challenge. A few strategies can make meals more palatable for those with particular tastes. Try hiding vegetables in sauces and casseroles, blending them into a smooth texture that becomes part of the dish. Pureed carrots can enhance the sweetness of a tomato sauce, while finely chopped spinach might go unnoticed in a lasagna. Offering a variety of options at each meal allows everyone to find something they enjoy. If one dish doesn't appeal, ensure there are side options that can stand alone, such as a simple green salad or roasted potatoes.

Family-friendly meals bring together the joy of cooking and the satisfaction of shared dining experiences. These strategies cater to diverse palates and promote healthy habits and family bonding. As you explore these meal ideas, remember that the goal is to create a welcoming environment where everyone feels included and excited about what's on their plate. In the next chapter, we will delve into case studies and success stories, showcasing the transformative power of the anti-inflammatory diet in real-life scenarios.

CHAPTER 10

SUCCESS STORIES

In health and wellness, stories of transformation can inspire and motivate like nothing else. Picture a garden in spring, where buds blossom into vibrant flowers, each unique yet universally beautiful. Similarly, personal journeys with the anti-inflammatory diet reveal profound changes, both seen and felt. These narratives are not just tales of dietary shifts; they are chronicles of resilience, showing how individuals from diverse backgrounds have harnessed the power of nutrition to rewrite their health destinies.

Consider the story of a young professional named Emily, who faced the debilitating grip of chronic fatigue. Her days blurred into a haze of exhaustion, each morning a battle against the invisible weight that sapped her energy. Despite her relentless drive and ambition, Emily found herself unable to perform at her best. It was a chance encounter with the anti-inflammatory diet that sparked hope. Gradually, as she embraced whole foods and mindful eating, Emily noticed a shift. Her energy levels began to rise, and she was no longer a scarce resource rationed throughout the day. Her mental clarity sharpened, transforming her work and personal life into realms of possibility.

Emily's journey illustrates the profound impact that dietary choices can have on one's vitality, offering a beacon of hope to those trapped in the cycle of fatigue.

Then there's Harold, a retiree who had resigned to a life constrained by aching joints and reduced mobility. The golden years, once envisioned as a chapter of exploration and leisure, seemed overshadowed by physical limitations. Yet, Harold's story took an unexpected turn. Encouraged by his family, he ventured into the world of anti-inflammatory eating. The changes were not immediate, but they were steady and undeniable. As Harold incorporated more fruits, vegetables, and omega-rich foods into his diet, his body responded. Joints that once creaked with every movement now supported him with newfound ease. Activities that had become distant memories—like gardening and walking in the park—became part of his daily routine again. Harold's transformation wasn't just physical; it infused his life with renewed joy and purpose.

These stories, while unique, share common threads of emotional and physical metamorphosis. For Emily and Harold, the journey began with uncertainty and required perseverance. The initial dietary adjustments posed challenges, from cravings for familiar comforts to navigating social settings. Yet, with each small victory —a morning without fatigue, a painless stroll—they found motivation to continue. The emotional shifts were equally significant. Enhanced mood and reduced anxiety became constants, replacing the shadows of doubt and frustration that once lingered. The anti-inflammatory diet became more than a regimen; it was a catalyst for holistic well-being, proving that change, while daunting, is within reach.

The obstacles faced by Emily and Harold resonate with many. The struggle to adapt to new eating patterns, the desire for immediate results, and the pressure of maintaining consistency are familiar to anyone who has embarked on a journey of transformation. Yet, it is through these challenges that triumph is forged. The key lies in celebrating every small milestone and finding strength in the incremental changes. For Emily, it was the first day she didn't need an afternoon nap, and for Harold, it was the joy of walking without pain. Though seemingly mundane, these moments are profound markers of progress, fueling the resolve to continue.

Consider creating a personal transformation timeline. Document each milestone, from the first day of the diet to notable changes in energy, mood, and physical abilities. Visualizing progress can reinforce motivation and highlight the transformative power of the anti-inflammatory diet.

As you read these stories, may you find a sense of connection and possibility. Whether you identify with Emily's fatigue or Harold's quest for mobility, know you are not alone. These tales are reminders that transformation is possible at any stage of life. They echo the experiences of countless others who have walked similar paths, armed with determination and guided by the principles of an anti-inflammatory lifestyle. Through their journeys, you are invited to reflect on your own, to embrace the potential for change, and to step boldly toward a healthier, more vibrant future.

10.1 OVERCOMING CHRONIC ILLNESS WITH DIET

In the world of chronic illness, where symptoms often dictate the rhythm of life, dietary interventions have emerged as a beacon of hope. Take the story of Margaret, a middle-aged woman who lived with arthritis. For years, she endured the constant ache of swelling joints, each movement a reminder of her condition. Traditional treatments brought limited relief, so Margaret sought alternatives. Guided by a nutritionist, she embarked on an anti-inflammatory diet. The transformation was gradual yet profound. Eliminating trigger foods like processed meats and refined sugars, Margaret introduced a colorful array of fruits, vegetables, and omega- 3-rich fish into her meals. These changes did more than soothe her symptoms; they revitalized her entire being. As weeks turned into months, the stiffness in her joints diminished, and her mobility improved. Margaret's story exemplifies the power of dietary choices in managing chronic conditions, offering a testament to the tangible benefits of embracing nutrient-rich foods.

Consider also the journey of David, a man diagnosed with Crohn's disease— a condition marked by inflammation of the digestive tract. His life was punctuated by periods of intense discomfort and dietary restrictions that seemed to offer little respite. Yet, through careful dietary adjustments, David found a path to remission. Working closely with healthcare providers, he identified and systematically eliminated foods exacerbating his symptoms. Wheat and dairy, once staples, were replaced by gut-friendly alternatives like quinoa and almond milk. David's diet became a tapestry of anti-inflammatory ingredients, from leafy greens to turmeric-spiced dishes. His commitment to this new way of eating was unwavering, and the results were nothing short of remarkable. Over time, his symptoms abated, and he gained a newfound sense of control over his health. David's experience highlights the critical role that tailored dietary strategies can play in managing and alleviating the symptoms of chronic illnesses.

Central to these stories is the collaboration with healthcare professionals. Margaret and David recognized the importance of guidance from nutritionists and doctors, ensuring their dietary changes complement existing treatments. Regular consultations allowed for adjustments to medication and nutritional plans, creating a holistic approach to health management. This collaboration was vital in achieving the best outcomes, as it provided a framework within which dietary interventions could thrive. For Margaret, this meant incorporating specific anti- inflammatory supplements under her doctor's supervision, enhancing the effects of her diet. For David, it involved ongoing monitoring of his inflammatory markers, ensuring that his nutritional choices effectively supported his remission. These partnerships underscore the value of integrating professional expertise into personal health journeys, paving the way for informed and effective dietary interventions.

Measurable health outcomes substantiate the impact of these dietary changes. In their blood tests, Margaret and David documented significant decreases in inflammatory markers, such as C-reactive protein (CRP). These markers, often used to gauge inflammation in the body, provided tangible evidence of the positive effects of their dietary choices. Additionally, quality of life scores, which assess individuals' overall well-being and day-to-day functionality, showed marked improvements. For Margaret, this translated into being able to engage in activities she had long forsaken, like gardening and hiking. David, too, experienced an uplift in his daily life, enjoying meals without the looming fear of discomfort. These metrics are powerful reminders of dietary changes' potential in managing chronic illnesses, offering hope and inspiration to others navigating similar paths.

While distinct, these stories of Margaret and David share a common theme: the transformative potential of diet in managing chronic conditions. They illustrate how carefully selecting foods can alleviate symptoms and enhance quality of life, providing a roadmap for those seeking to reclaim their health. Through collaboration with healthcare providers and a commitment to dietary adjustments, individuals like Margaret and David demonstrate that change is possible, even in the face of chronic illness. Their experiences testify to thoughtful nutrition's profound impact, offering a beacon of hope for others on similar journeys.

10.2 LONG-TERM HEALTH IMPROVEMENTS

In the tapestry of life, where each thread represents a choice or habit, some individuals have woven stories of lasting health changes through the anti-inflammatory diet. These narratives stretch across years, illustrating how sustained efforts can yield profound results. Take, for instance, the story of James, who embarked on a decade-long commitment to healthier living. James initially struggled to balance work and personal life, often resorting to fast food and neglecting physical activity. However, he gradually embraced meal planning and prepared wholesome meals at home. By focusing on foods rich in nutrients and low in inflammatory potential, James noticed a steady improvement in his vitality. His transformation wasn't overnight; it was a testament to persistence and adaptability. Over time, he incorporated regular exercise and stress management practices, such as yoga and meditation, which became integral to his routine. These changes improved his physical health and enhanced his emotional wellbeing, creating a balanced and fulfilling life.

Similarly, the Rivera family offers a compelling example of collective commitment to health. Motivated to improve their lifestyle, they adopted an anti-inflammatory diet together. This decision began a new chapter, where family meals became opportunities for connection and learning. They experimented with new recipes, incorporating colorful vegetables, lean proteins, and healthy fats into their meals. Each family member contributed by choosing recipes, grocery shopping, or cooking. This collaborative approach fostered a sense of unity and shared purpose. Over the years, the Rivera family achieved better health markers and developed a deeper bond. Their story underscores the power of community and shared goals in sustaining long-term health improvements.

For individuals like James and families like the Riveras, sustainable lifestyle changes have been vital in maintaining their health gains. Consistent meal planning and preparation ensure they have control over their food choices, avoiding the pitfalls of convenience foods laden with unhealthy ingredients. Regular physical activity, whether through structured exercise or active hobbies, supports the body's resilience against inflammation. Stress management practices, tailored to their preferences, provide a sanctuary amidst life's demands, mitigating the impact of stress on their health. These habits, cultivated over time, form a robust foundation for well- being, enabling them to navigate life's challenges with confidence and vigor.

Staying motivated in the long term often requires setting new health goals and challenges. James found inspiration in tracking his progress, using milestones to celebrate achievements and identify areas for growth. For the Riveras, the journey became about continuous learning, exploring new cuisines, and adapting dietary choices to keep meals exciting and relevant. This proactive approach ensures their lifestyle remains dynamic and aligned with their evolving needs. They recognize that health is a journey, not a destination, and remain open to new ideas and approaches that enhance their well-being.

The lessons learned from these stories offer valuable insights for anyone seeking long-term health improvements. Persistence and patience are paramount; change takes time, and setbacks are part of the process. Celebrating progress, no matter how small, reinforces positive behaviors and keeps motivation alive. Embracing a mindset of curiosity and adaptability allows for growth and resilience, enabling individuals to thrive amidst change. These narratives remind us that the path to health is a personal and evolving journey, shaped by choices and reinforced by community and support. As you reflect on these stories, consider how their lessons might inspire your own health journey, guiding you toward a life of vitality and fulfillment.

10.3 STORIES OF WEIGHT MANAGEMENT SUCCESS

In the tapestry of life, our relationship with food and body image can often be tangled with emotions and societal expectations. For many, achieving and maintaining a healthy weight is not just a physical battle but also an emotional one. Meet Alex, a young adult who faced the daunting challenge of obesity. Growing up, Alex found comfort in food, a solace that gradually became a burden. The weight crept up slowly, each pound adding to the physical and emotional strain. After a wake-up call during a routine check-up, Alex decided to transform his lifestyle with an anti-inflammatory diet. By focusing on portion control and embracing mindful eating, he began to see results. Meals became moments of nourishment rather than indulgence. Low- calorie, nutrient-dense foods like leafy greens and lean proteins became staples. Over time, Alex's weight decreased, and with it, his confidence grew. Alex's success is measured not just in lost pounds but in the newfound zest for life he discovered along the way.

CHAPTER 11

TRACKING PROGRESS AND STAYING MOTIVATED

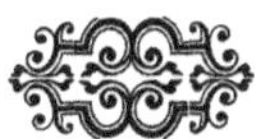

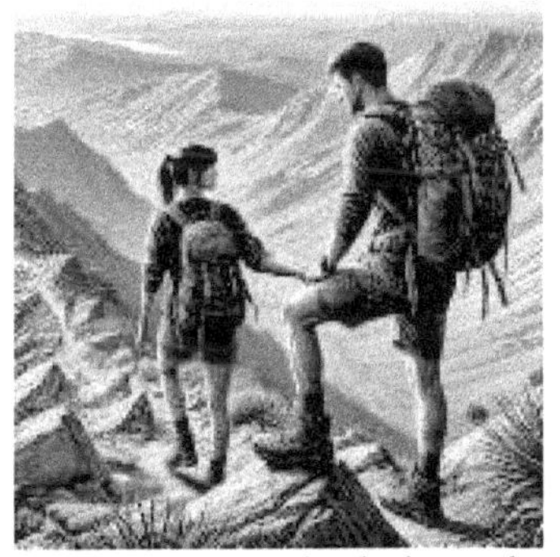For Sarah, a mother navigating the postpartum period, the goal was to regain her pre- pregnancy weight. Juggling the demands of a newborn with the desire to feel like herself again, she turned to the anti-inflammatory diet as a path to renewal. Sarah's journey involved integrating foods rich in anti-inflammatory properties, such as berries, nuts, and whole grains. These foods supported her weight loss and provided the energy she needed to keep up with her active toddler. Portion control played a crucial role, helping her manage cravings and stay on track. Sarah also found solace in mindful eating practices, savoring each bite and listening to her body's hunger and fullness signals. As her body transformed, her self-esteem soared, reinforcing that weight management is as much about mental well-being as physical change.

The positive ripple effects of weight management extend far beyond the numbers on a scale. Both Alex and Sarah experienced a profound boost in self-esteem and confidence. With each milestone reached, their belief in their ability to effect change grew stronger. Physical performance also improved significantly. Alex, once winded by a short walk, now found joy in regular runs, each stride a testament to his newfound stamina. Sarah also discovered a love for yoga, a practice that strengthened her body and connected her to a community of supportive individuals. These activities, once daunting, became sources of joy and fulfillment, illustrating the holistic benefits of a healthier weight.

Setting realistic and attainable goals is vital for those inspired by these stories. Start by identifying small, actionable steps that align with your lifestyle. It could be incorporating one new vegetable into your weekly meals or committing to a daily walk around the block. Finding enjoyable forms of physical activity is equally important. Exercise should not feel like a chore but rather a celebration of movement. Whether it's dancing, swimming, or hiking, the goal is to move in ways that bring happiness. Embrace the journey with patience and kindness towards yourself, knowing that each step forward is a victory in its own right.

Inspiration often comes from those who have walked the path before us. Let Alex and Sarah's stories be a reminder that weight management is within reach. Their journeys highlight the power of the anti-inflammatory diet as a tool not only for physical transformation but also for enhancing overall well-being. As you consider your own path, remember that change is possible and sustainable with dedication, support, and the right strategies. Their experiences offer a glimpse into the possibilities that await when you take that first step towards a healthier, more vibrant life.

Chapter 10 concludes with these stories of transformation, illustrating the profound impact of the anti-inflammatory diet on weight management and overall well-being. These narratives bridge the next chapter, where we explore how to stay motivated and track your progress.

Imagine setting off on an expedition, armed with a map and compass, ready to navigate the terrain ahead. Much like this journey, your health goals require careful planning and direction. The path to wellness through an anti-inflammatory diet is no different. Here, the map is your goals, and the compass is your motivation. Setting clear, achievable goals is your guiding light, providing the momentum you need to stay the course. Without them, it's like wandering through a forest without a trail, where progress feels elusive and efforts scattered. Establishing goals creates a structured path that leads you to tangible results and sustained motivation.

Understanding the distinction between short-term and long-term goals is vital for goal setting. Short-term goals are the stepping stones that keep you engaged and focused. They might include weekly meal planning or incorporating a new anti-inflammatory recipe each week. These goals are bite-sized and actionable, making them attainable and rewarding. On the other hand, long-term goals are the overarching vision, such as reducing inflammation markers or achieving a specific weight target over several months. Aligning these goals with your personal values ensures they resonate deeply, providing intrinsic motivation and a sense of purpose. When your goals reflect what truly matters to you, they're more likely to withstand challenges and distractions.

Creating SMART goals transforms aspirations into actionable steps. The SMART framework— Specific, Measurable, Achievable, Relevant, and Time-bound—is a powerful tool in this process. A specific goal might involve preparing two anti-inflammatory meals each day. Measurable means tracking your progress by noting how many days you achieve this weekly goal. Achievable ensures the goal is within reach, considering your current lifestyle and resources. Relevance ties the goal to your broader health objectives, ensuring it contributes meaningfully to your journey. Finally, making the goal time-bound sets a deadline, such as achieving this routine within a month, adding urgency and focus. By adhering to the SMART principles, your goals become clear roadmaps, guiding your efforts and measuring your achievements.

Breaking down your goals into smaller milestones makes progress more manageable and rewarding. Each milestone represents a mini-victory, a moment to pause and celebrate how far you've come. These could be as simple as successfully switching to whole grains for a week or incorporating more vegetables into your daily meals. Identifying key milestones in your dietary changes helps keep motivation high, as you can see tangible evidence of your efforts translating into progress. Celebrating these achievements, no matter how small, reinforces your commitment and boosts your confidence, reminding you that each step forward is a step towards better health.

Practical templates and worksheets can be invaluable in assisting with goal setting. A weekly goal-setting worksheet encourages you to outline your objectives, track your efforts, and reflect on your progress. This visual representation of your journey offers clarity and keeps you accountable. Progress charts further enhance this process, providing a snapshot of your achievements over time. By charting your progress, you can identify patterns, recognize successes, and adjust your strategy. These tools organize your efforts and motivate you, reminding you of your dedication and the positive changes you're making.

Goal-Setting Worksheet

Consider using a goal-setting worksheet to map out your health objectives. Include sections for:

- Short-term and long-term goals
- SMART criteria for each goal
- Weekly milestones
- Reflections on progress and adjustments needed

This exercise empowers you to take control, offering a structured approach to achieving your health aspirations.

11.1 USING TECHNOLOGY TO TRACK YOUR JOURNEY

In today's digital age, technology offers many tools that can transform how you monitor your dietary habits and lifestyle changes. Picture your smartphone or smartwatch as a gadget and a personal health assistant ready to guide you toward wellness. Nutrition tracking apps like MyFitnessPal have become indispensable for many, offering the ability to log meals, count calories, and analyze nutrient intake with ease. These apps provide detailed insights into your eating patterns, helping you identify areas that need adjustment. Meanwhile, wearable fitness trackers like Fitbit or Garmin devices keep tabs on your physical activity, heart rate, and sleep patterns. They constantly remind you of your goals, nudging you to move more and rest adequately.

The benefits of using technology for tracking go beyond mere data collection. They help you understand the intricate patterns of your lifestyle, revealing insights that might otherwise go unnoticed. By analyzing your dietary intake, you can ensure your meals are balanced, providing all the essential nutrients your body needs. This analysis can highlight any deficiencies or excesses in your diet, enabling you to make informed adjustments. Monitoring your physical activity levels is equally important. It allows you to assess whether you're meeting your fitness goals and identify opportunities to incorporate more movement into your daily routine. This holistic view of your habits empowers you to take control of your health, making informed decisions backed by real-time data.

To maximize the benefits of technology, consider implementing a few practical strategies. Start by setting reminders to log your meals and activities consistently. These reminders can help establish a routine, making tracking a seamless part of your day. Periodically review weekly summaries provided by the apps. These overviews offer valuable insights into your progress, helping you recognize patterns and areas for improvement. You can quickly identify trends and make necessary changes by visualizing your habits. Regular reviews keep you engaged with your health journey and help you stay on track with your goals.

While technology offers incredible advantages, addressing privacy and data concerns is crucial. With the increasing reliance on apps and devices, safeguarding your personal information becomes paramount. When selecting apps, prioritize those with strong privacy policies. These policies should clearly outline how your data is collected, stored, and used. Understanding data- sharing settings is also essential. Some apps may share your information with third parties, so reviewing and adjusting these settings according to your comfort level is necessary. By taking these precautions, you can enjoy the benefits of technology while ensuring your data remains secure. Consider using a privacy checklist to evaluate apps before downloading. Include a review of the privacy policy, data and permission sharing settings. This checklist empowers you to make informed decisions about app security, ensuring a safe and beneficial tracking experience.

11.2 CELEBRATING SMALL WINS

As you navigate the path of dietary changes and lifestyle adjustments, it's easy to focus solely on future goals and overlook the victories. Yet, recognizing these small achievements is vital for maintaining motivation and building confidence. No matter how minor, each step contributes to a larger success. Acknowledging these moments can reinforce positive habits and keep your spirits high. Consider each small win a building block, laying a solid foundation for your health journey. By celebrating these incremental successes, you empower yourself to continue striving for more, knowing that progress is being made with each choice and action.

Finding creative ways to celebrate these achievements can align with your health goals, adding joy and satisfaction to the process. Rather than reaching for traditional rewards like indulgent foods, think outside the box. Treat yourself to a healthy cooking class to learn new recipes and techniques, enriching your culinary skills while staying true to your dietary changes.

Alternatively, consider non-food-related treats like a relaxing spa day or a new book that inspires you. These celebrations serve as a reminder that the journey to better health is not just about sacrifice but also about enjoyment and self-care. They provide moments of reflection and joy, reinforcing the idea that progress is worth celebrating.

Reflection plays a crucial role in recognizing growth and understanding the impact of your efforts. Journaling about personal achievements allows you to document your experiences, thoughts, and emotions, creating a tangible record of your progress. It offers a space to reflect on challenges overcome and lessons learned, fostering a deeper connection to your goals.

Sharing your progress with friends or family adds a communal aspect to your journey. It invites support and encouragement, allowing others to celebrate your successes with you. This act of sharing strengthens bonds and serves as an external acknowledgment of your hard work, enhancing your sense of accomplishment and motivation.

Positive reinforcement is a powerful tool in sustaining motivation and commitment. Creating a visual progress board can constantly remind you of your achievements and goals. Use it to display milestones reached, motivational quotes, and images that inspire you. This visual representation is a daily source of encouragement, reminding you of your capabilities and progress. Additionally, incorporating affirmations into your routine can boost self-esteem and reinforce positive thinking. Simple statements like "I am capable of change" or "I celebrate my progress" can shift your mindset, helping you focus on the positive aspects of your journey.

When repeated regularly, these affirmations can enhance your confidence and strengthen your resolve, creating a cycle of positivity that propels you forward.

Affirmation Creation Exercise

Spend a few moments crafting personal affirmations that resonate with your health goals. Write them down and place them somewhere visible, such as your bathroom mirror or workspace.

Recite them daily to reinforce your commitment and mindset.

How to Create Self-Affirmations

Self-affirmations are positive statements you say to yourself to build confidence, focus on your strengths, and push back against negative thoughts. Think of them as little reminders to help you stay grounded

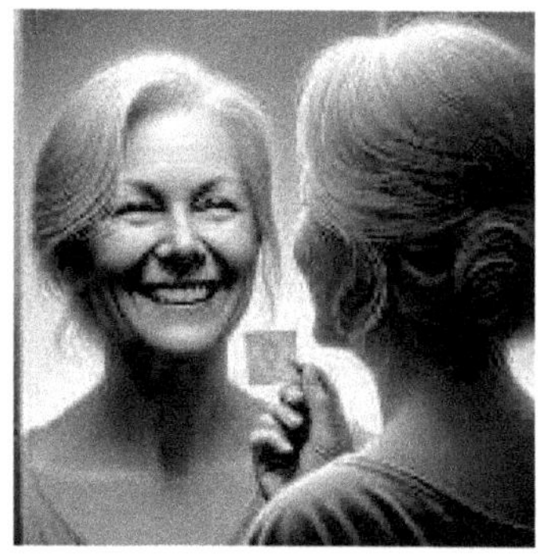

and motivated. The great thing is, they're personal—you create affirmations that feel meaningful to you and reflect the person you want to be.

Start With What You Need

Think about what's going on in your life right now. Are there areas where you feel stuck, unsure, or down on yourself? Maybe you're feeling nervous about a new job, struggling with self-doubt, or trying to build better habits. Use this as a starting point. For example, if you're feeling overwhelmed, try something like, "I am calm and capable of handling what comes my way."

Keep It Positive and Present

When making affirmations, focus on what you want, not what you don't. Instead of saying, "I won't fail," go for something like, "I have what it takes to succeed." Always use positive language and keep it in the present tense, like it's already true. Short and simple affirmations are easier to remember and more impactful when you repeat them.

Make It a Daily Habit

For affirmations to work, you need to use them regularly. Say them to yourself in the mirror, write them in a journal, or just think them in your head during quiet moments. The more you repeat them, the more they'll stick. Try pairing them with actions, too. For instance, if your affirmation is, "I take care of my health," follow it up with small steps like drinking more water or stretching.

Adjust as You Go

Over time, you might notice your affirmations helping you feel more confident or positive. That's great! Celebrate those little wins and adjust your affirmations if your goals change. The key is to keep them meaningful and relevant to where you're at in life. Self-affirmations are all about giving yourself a boost and staying kind to yourself along the way

11.3 BUILDING A SUPPORTIVE COMMUNITY

Imagine walking into a room filled with people who share your aspirations and challenges. This is the essence of a supportive community. Having a network of like-minded individuals can be transformative when embarking on dietary and lifestyle changes. Community support offers shared experiences and encouragement, creating a space to exchange insights, celebrate progress, and find solace in knowing you're not alone. Accountability is another powerful aspect of a community. When others know your goals, they can offer gentle reminders and motivation to keep you on track, making it easier to maintain your commitments even when the going gets tough. The collective wisdom of a group can provide solutions and perspectives that you might not have considered, enriching your journey and enhancing your resilience.

Finding the right support group begins with exploring various platforms and opportunities. Online forums and social media groups dedicated to health, wellness, and specific dietary interests are abundant and accessible. These virtual spaces allow you to connect with individuals from diverse backgrounds, sharing tips, recipes, and motivational stories. They provide a sense of belonging and can be particularly beneficial if you live in a remote area or have a busy schedule. Local meetups and community classes offer a more personal touch, providing face-to- face interaction and the chance to build deeper connections. Whether it's a cooking class focused on anti-inflammatory meals or a walking group that meets weekly, these gatherings foster camaraderie and support. They create an environment where you can learn together, share successes, and even find accountability partners to help you stay committed to your goals.

Active participation in these communities is crucial for reaping their full benefits. Engage with the group by joining challenges or events that promote healthy habits. These activities provide structure and motivation and make the process enjoyable and rewarding. Sharing your own recipes and success stories can inspire others and create a sense of reciprocity, where everyone contributes to and benefits from the collective knowledge. This exchange of ideas and experiences strengthens the community, making it a vibrant and supportive network.

Additionally, offering encouragement to others can reinforce your own commitment as you become both a student and a teacher in the shared pursuit of wellness.

Navigating community dynamics requires sensitivity and respect, mainly when differing opinions arise. It's essential to approach discussions openly, recognizing that everyone is on their path and may have different methods and beliefs. Respectful dialogue fosters a positive atmosphere where diverse perspectives coexist and enrich the group's overall experience. At times, maintaining focus on your personal goals amidst group dynamics can be challenging. It's easy to get swept up in the enthusiasm or opinions of others, but grounding yourself in your objectives is vital. Regularly revisiting your goals and reminding yourself of your motivations can help you stay centered. This balance allows you to benefit from the community's support while staying true to your path.

As you integrate these practices into your routine, the power of community support becomes evident. The shared journey of growth and change is enriched by the collective energy and wisdom of those around you. By participating in these networks, you not only enhance your own experience but also contribute to a culture of support and encouragement. This chapter of your health journey highlights the importance of connection, illustrating how community engagement can create a ripple effect of positive change. As you move forward, remember that embracing the support of others is not a sign of weakness but a source of strength. Together, we can achieve more than we ever could alone.

CONCLUSION

As we reach the end of this journey together, let's take a moment to reflect on the core concepts that have guided us. We've delved into the intricate world of inflammation, understanding how it acts as a guardian and, when unchecked, a potential foe to our well-being. Throughout this book, we have explored the transformative power of an anti-inflammatory diet. Choosing foods rich in nutrients and antioxidants can support your body's natural healing processes and manage chronic conditions more effectively. This holistic approach to health isn't just about what you eat—it's about integrating lifestyle changes that promote overall wellness.

My vision for this book has always been clear: to empower you with knowledge and practical tools to navigate and manage inflammation naturally. It's about enabling you to make informed dietary and lifestyle choices that can lead to lasting health improvements. In doing so, I hope that you feel confident in taking control of your health journey, armed with the insights and strategies we've discussed.

Among the key takeaways, we've highlighted the transformative power of whole, nutrient-dense foods as the foundation for reducing inflammation and enhancing overall vitality. Understanding and identifying inflammatory triggers empowers you to make smarter, more informed choices that align with your health goals. Beyond diet, embracing holistic practices—like managing stress, staying active, and cultivating balance—ensures that your approach to well-being is both comprehensive and sustainable. Together, these steps pave the way for a healthier, more resilient you, allowing you to take control of your health and thrive with energy, purpose, and clarity.

BONUS RECIPE BOOK

ANTI-INFLAMMATORY MEALS UNDER 30 MINUTES

THE ANTI-INFLAMMATORY BREAKFAST

Imagine the morning sun rising, marking the start of a new day full of possibilities. You're seeking something quick, nourishing, and satisfying—a meal that energizes you and sets the tone for the hours ahead. This is where the art of crafting a quick and easy breakfast comes into play, with recipes designed to seamlessly fit into your morning routine while embracing the 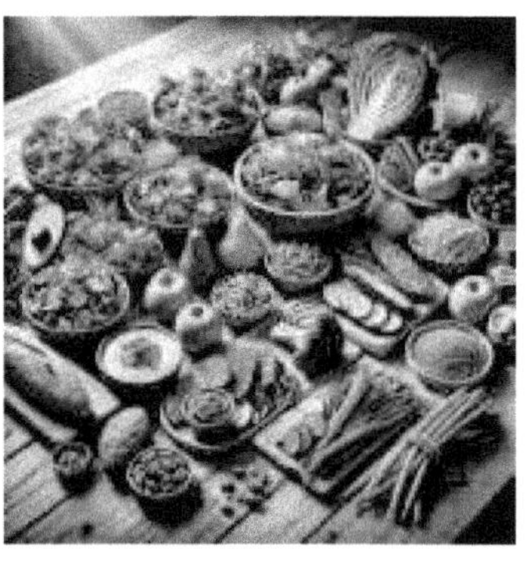 anti- inflammatory principles we've explored. In this chapter, you'll find recipes that are not only swift to prepare but also bursting with flavors and nutrients to fuel your day and support your health goals.

Overnight Oats with Berries and Almond Butter

Start your morning off right with Overnight Oats with Berries and Almond Butter, a breakfast that's as convenient as it is nutritious. This make-ahead meal combines the creamy texture of oats with the natural sweetness of fresh berries and the richness of almond butter. Packed with fiber, healthy fats, and antioxidants, it provides sustained energy to fuel your day while supporting your anti-inflammatory goals.

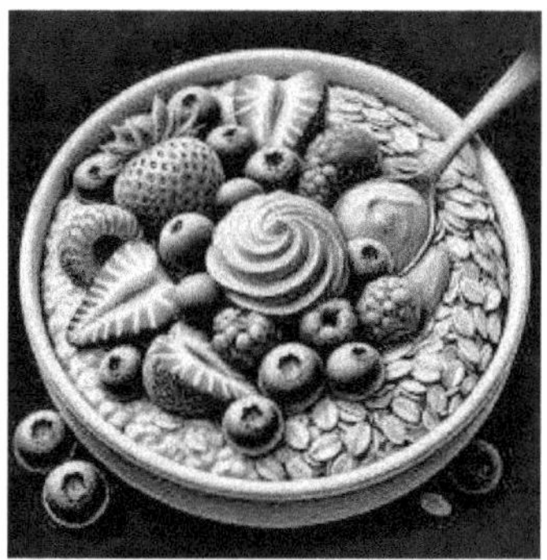

Perfect for busy mornings, this recipe requires minimal effort yet delivers maximum flavor and nourishment, making it a go-to option for a healthy and satisfying start to your day.

Nutritional Information (Per Serving):

- Calories: 250
- Protein: 6g
- Fat: 9g
- Carbohydrates: 35g
- Fiber: 8g
- Vitamin C: 10% DV
- Iron: 10% DV
- Calcium: 15% DV

Ingredients:

- ½ cup rolled oats
- ½ cup almond milk
- tablespoon chia seeds
- ¼ cup mixed fresh berries
- teaspoon almond butter

Instructions:

- Combine oats, almond milk, and chia seeds in a jar or bowl. Stir well. Cover and refrigerate overnight. Top with fresh berries and a drizzle of
- almond butter before serving.

Green Smoothie Bowl

Kickstart your morning with a vibrant Green Smoothie Bowl, packed with nutrient-rich ingredients to fuel your day. The creamy green base, made with spinach and avocado, is complemented by a colorful array of toppings like bananas, fresh berries, and crunchy chia seeds. This anti-inflammatory breakfast provides a boost of antioxidants, fiber, and healthy fats, delivering both nutrition and flavor in every spoonful.

Nutritional Information (Per Serving):

- Calories: 280
- Protein: 6g
- Fat: 15g
- Carbohydrates: 30g
- Fiber: 7g
- Vitamin A: 50% DV
- Vitamin C: 70% DV
- Iron: 10% DV
- Calcium: 15% DV

Ingredients:

- frozen banana
- cup spinach
- ½ avocado
- 1 cup unsweetened almond milk
- Toppings: ¼ cup fresh berries, 1 teaspoon chia seeds, 2 tablespoons sliced almonds

Instructions:

- Blend Smoothie Base: Blend the banana, spinach, avocado, and almond milk until smooth and creamy.

- Assemble Bowl: Pour the smoothie into a bowl and arrange the toppings on top.
- Serve: Enjoy immediately with a spoon for a refreshing start to your day.

Whole-Grain Pancakes with Berries and Maple Syrup

Start your day with a comforting and wholesome breakfast: WholeGrain Pancakes with Berries and Maple Syrup. These pancakes are light, fluffy, and packed with fiber and nutrients, thanks to the wholegrain flour. Topped with fresh berries and a drizzle of pure maple syrup, they're both satisfying and nourishing, offering a perfect balance of flavor and anti-inflammatory goodness.

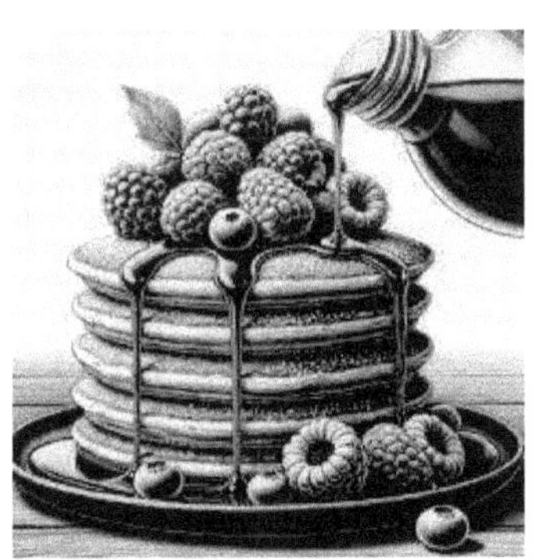

Nutritional Information (Per Serving, Makes 4 Pancakes):

- Calories: 250
- Protein: 7g Fat: 4g
- Carbohydrates: 48g
- Fiber: 6g
- Vitamin C: 20% DV
- Iron: 15% DV
- Calcium: 12% DV

Ingredients:

- cup whole-grain flour
- teaspoon baking powder
- 1 tablespoon honey or maple syrup
- 1 egg (or flaxseed egg for a vegan option)
- ¾ cup almond milk
- ¼ teaspoon vanilla extract
- Toppings: ½ cup mixed berries, 1 tablespoon pure maple syrup

Instructions:

- Prepare the Batter: In a bowl, mix the flour and baking powder. In another bowl, whisk the egg, almond milk, honey, and vanilla. Gradually combine the wet and dry ingredients until smooth.
- Cook Pancakes: Heat a non-stick skillet over medium heat. Pour ¼ cup of batter onto the skillet and cook until bubbles form on the surface, then flip and cook until golden brown. Repeat with remaining batter.
- Serve: Stack pancakes on a plate, top with fresh berries, and drizzle with maple syrup.

Avocado Toast with Egg

Simple, satisfying, and packed with nutrients, Avocado Toast with Egg is a perfect way to start your day. Creamy avocado spread on toasted whole-grain bread provides healthy fats and fiber, while a soft-boiled egg adds a boost of protein to keep you energized. With just a sprinkle of red pepper flakes or your favorite seasoning, this breakfast is both delicious and anti-inflammatory.

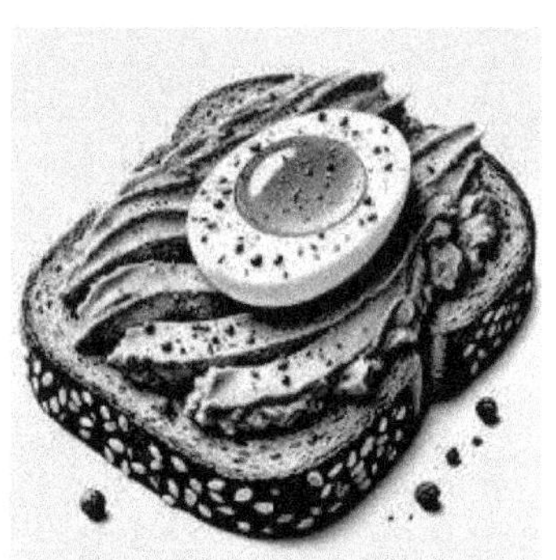

Nutritional Information (Per Serving):

- Calories: 220
- Protein: 10g
- Fat: 14g
- Carbohydrates: 16g
- Fiber: 6g
- Vitamin A: 8% DV
- Iron: 10% DV
- Calcium: 4% DV

Ingredients:

- slice whole-grain bread (toasted)
- ½ avocado (smashed)
- soft-boiled egg
- Pinch of red pepper flakes or salt and pepper

Instructions:
- Toast Bread: Toast the whole-grain bread until golden and crisp.

- Prepare Toppings: Spread smashed avocado evenly over the toast.
- Add Egg: Slice the soft-boiled egg and layer it on top of the avocado.
- Season: Sprinkle with red pepper flakes, salt, and pepper to taste.

Chia Seed Pudding with Berries

Elevate your breakfast with Chia Seed Pudding with Berries, a creamy and nutrient-packed dish that's as delicious as it is nourishing. Rich in omega-3s, fiber, and antioxidants, this make-ahead breakfast is perfect for busy mornings. Topped with fresh berries and a sprinkle of granola, it's a satisfying and anti-inflammatory way to start your day.

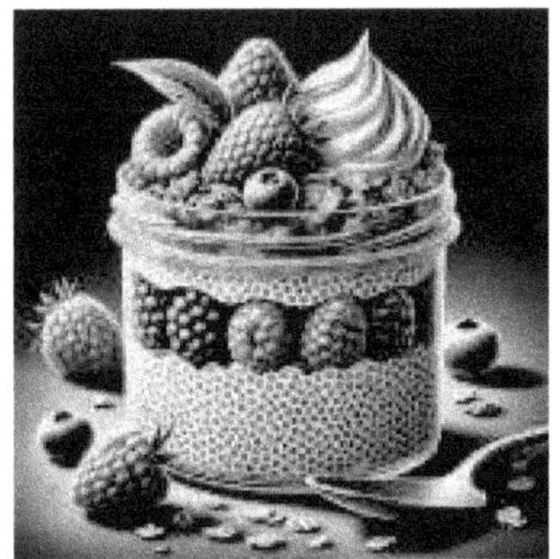

Nutritional Information (Per Serving, Makes 2 Servings):

- Calories: 180
- Protein: 6g
- Fat: 8g
- Carbohydrates: 22g
- Fiber: 10g
- Vitamin C: 20% DV
- Iron: 10% DV
- Calcium: 15% DV

Ingredients:

- 3 tablespoons chia seeds
- cup unsweetened almond milk
- teaspoon vanilla extract
- ½ cup fresh mixed berries
- tablespoons granola (optional for topping)

Instructions:

- Prepare Pudding: In a jar or bowl, combine chia seeds, almond milk, and vanilla extract. Stir well to prevent clumping.
- Refrigerate: Cover and refrigerate overnight or for at least 4 hours until the pudding thickens.
- Serve: Top with fresh berries and granola before serving.

Spinach and Vegetable Omelette

A hearty and nutrient-packed Spinach and Vegetable Omelette is the perfect way to kick off your morning. Packed with protein and vibrant vegetables, this savory dish offers a delicious blend of sautéed spinach, bell peppers, and onions, folded into fluffy eggs. This quick and anti- inflammatory breakfast will keep you energized and satisfied throughout your day.

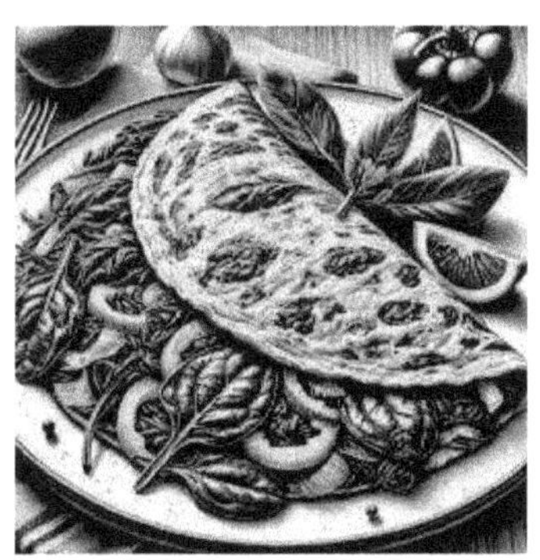

Nutritional Information (Per Serving):

- Calories: 200
- Protein: 12g
- Fat: 14g
- Carbohydrates: 6g
- Fiber: 2g
- Vitamin A: 60% DV
- Vitamin C: 50% DV
- Iron: 15% DV
- Calcium: 8% DV

Ingredients:

- 2 large eggs
- cup fresh spinach (chopped)
- ¼ cup diced bell peppers
- ¼ cup diced onions
- tablespoon olive oil or ghee
- Pinch of salt and pepper

Instructions:

- Sauté Vegetables: Heat olive oil in a non-stick skillet over medium heat. Add bell peppers, onions, and spinach, cooking until softened. Remove from the skillet and set aside.
- Prepare Omelette: Beat the eggs with a pinch of salt and pepper. Pour into the skillet and cook until the edges start to set.
- Add Filling: Place the sautéed vegetables on one side of the omelette. Fold the omelette over and cook for another minute.
- Serve: Slide onto a plate, garnish with fresh herbs, and enjoy.

Yogurt Parfait with Granola and Berries

Start your day with a delicious and nourishing Yogurt Parfait with Granola and Berries. This layered breakfast combines creamy yogurt, crunchy granola, and the natural sweetness of fresh berries for a balanced and energizing meal. Packed with protein, fiber, and antioxidants, this anti-inflammatory dish is as beautiful as it is wholesome.

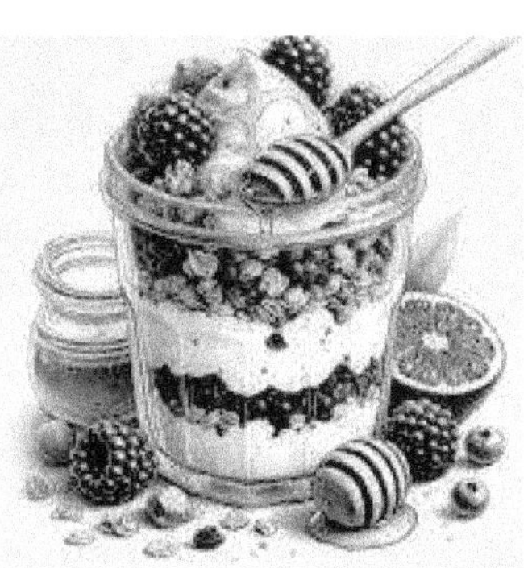

Nutritional Information (Per Serving, Makes 1 Serving):

- Calories: 220
- Protein: 12g
- Fat: 6g
- Carbohydrates:30g
- Fiber: 4g
- Vitamin C: 20% DV
- Calcium:15% DV
- Iron: 10% DV

Ingredients:

- cup plain Greek yogurt (or dairy-free yogurt for a vegan option)
- ½ cup granola (low-sugar or homemade)
- ½ cup fresh mixed berries
- teaspoon honey or maple syrup (optional)

Instructions:

- Layer Ingredients: In a glass or bowl, layer ⅓ of the yogurt at the bottom. Add ⅓ of the granola and ⅓ of the berries. Repeat Layers: Continue layering until all ingredients are used, finishing with berries on top.
- Optional Sweetener: Drizzle with honey or maple syrup for added sweetness.
- Serve: Enjoy immediately or refrigerate for up to 1 hour before serving.

Sweet Potato Breakfast Bowl

Transform your morning routine with this warm and nourishing Sweet Potato Breakfast Bowl. Packed with the natural sweetness of mashed sweet potatoes and topped with creamy almond butter, bananas, and crunchy granola, this dish is both comforting and nutritious. It's rich in fiber, vitamins, and healthy fats, making it an anti-inflammatory breakfast that fuels your day with wholesome energy.

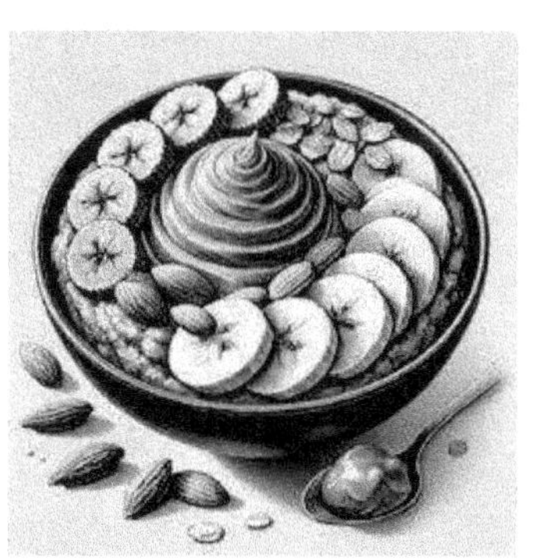

Nutritional Information (Per Serving, Makes 1 Serving):

- Calories: 280
- Protein: 5g
- Fat: 8g
- Carbohydrates: 50g
- Fiber: 7g
- Vitamin A: 150% DV
- Vitamin C: 20% DV
- Calcium: 8% DV
- Iron: 10% DV

Ingredients:

- medium sweet potato (roasted and mashed)
- 1 tablespoon almond butter
- ½ banana (sliced)
- 2 tablespoons granola
- Optional: pinch of cinnamon or nutmeg

Instructions:

- Prepare Sweet Potato: Roast or microwave the sweet potato until soft. Mash in a bowl.
- Add Toppings: Drizzle almond butter over the mashed sweet potato. Top with sliced bananas and granola. Optional Seasoning: Sprinkle with a pinch of cinnamon or nutmeg for added warmth and flavor.
- Serve: Enjoy warm for a cozy and satisfying start to your day.

Baked Almond Oatmeal

Warm, hearty, and delightfully satisfying, Baked Almond Oatmeal is a breakfast that feels like a treat while delivering excellent nutrition.

Made with wholesome oats and topped with sliced almonds and a drizzle of honey, this dish provides sustained energy and anti-inflammatory benefits. Perfect for a leisurely morning or meal-prepped in advance, it's a versatile and nourishing way to start your day.

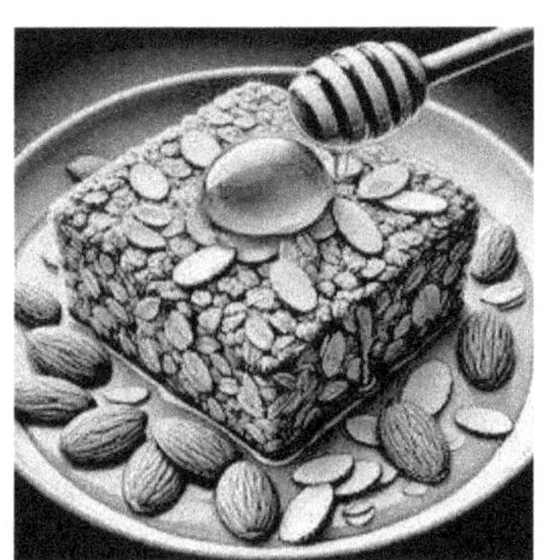

Nutritional Information (Per Serving, Makes 4 Servings):

- Calories: 220
- Protein: 5g
- Fat: 6g
- Carbohydrates: 36g
- Fiber: 5g
- Vitamin E: 10% DV
- Calcium: 15% DV
- Iron: 8% DV

Ingredients:

- cup rolled oats 1 cup almond milk
- tablespoon honey (or maple syrup)
- 1 teaspoon vanilla extract
- ½ teaspoon cinnamon
- ¼ cup sliced almonds

Instructions:

- Prepare the Mixture: Preheat the oven to 350°F (175°C). In a bowl, mix rolled oats, almond milk, honey, vanilla extract, and cinnamon.
- Assemble: Pour the mixture into a greased baking dish.
- Sprinkle sliced almonds on top.
- Bake: Bake for 20–25 minutes or until the top is golden and set.
- Serve: Slice into portions and enjoy warm. Add an extra drizzle of honey if desired.

Scrambled Eggs with Spinach and Avocado

Kickstart your morning with a protein-packed and nutrient-dense breakfast: Scrambled Eggs with Spinach and Avocado. The creamy avocado pairs beautifully with fluffy scrambled eggs and nutrient-rich spinach, creating a wholesome dish that's easy to prepare and perfect for an anti-inflammatory diet.

Nutritional Information (Per Serving, Makes 1 Serving):

- Calories: 230
- Protein: 12g
- Fat: 18g
- Carbohydrates: 6g
- Fiber: 3g
- Vitamin A: 50% DV
- Iron: 15% DV
- Calcium: 8% DV

Ingredients:

- 2 large eggs
- cup fresh spinach (chopped)
- ½ avocado (sliced)
- teaspoon olive oil
- Pinch of salt and pepper

Instructions:

- Cook Spinach: Heat olive oil in a skillet over medium heat.
- Add spinach and sauté until wilted.
- Scramble Eggs: Whisk the eggs with a pinch of salt and pepper. Pour into the skillet and cook, stirring gently, until softly set.

- Assemble: Plate the scrambled eggs with the spinach and top with avocado slices.
- Serve: Enjoy warm for a balanced and energizing start to your day.

Breakfast Burrito

Elevate your mornings with a wholesome Breakfast Burrito filled with scrambled eggs, black beans, sautéed peppers, and spinach. Wrapped in a whole-grain tortilla, this hearty breakfast delivers a balance of protein, fiber, and nutrients to fuel your day. Perfect for on-the-go mornings or a sit-down meal, this anti-inflammatory option is both satisfying and delicious.

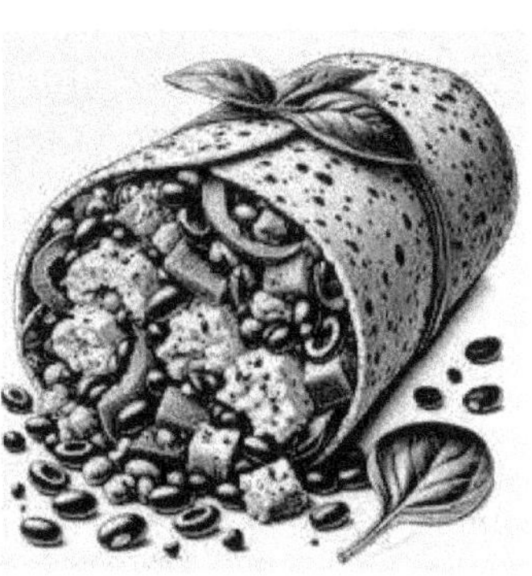

Nutritional Information (Per Serving, Makes 1 Serving):

- Calories: 300
- Protein: 15g
- Fat: 10g
- Carbohydrates: 35g
  Fiber: 7g
- Vitamin C: 40% DV
- Iron: 12% DV
- Calcium: 10% DV

Ingredients:

- 1 whole-grain tortilla
- 2 large eggs
- ¼ cup black beans (rinsed and drained)
- ¼ cup diced bell peppers
- cup fresh spinach (chopped)
- teaspoon olive oil
- Pinch of salt and pepper

Instructions:

- Sauté Vegetables: Heat olive oil in a skillet over medium heat. Add bell peppers and spinach, cooking until softened. Set aside.
- Scramble Eggs: Whisk eggs with salt and pepper. Pour into the skillet and cook until scrambled.
- Assemble Burrito: Warm the tortilla and layer the scrambled eggs, black beans, and sautéed vegetables in the center.
- Wrap and Serve: Fold the sides of the tortilla over the filling and roll tightly. Serve warm.

Banana Protein Pancakes

Start your morning with a stack of Banana Protein Pancakes, a nutrient-rich and delicious way to fuel your day. Made with ripe bananas and a boost of protein, these pancakes are fluffy, naturally sweet, and perfect for an anti-inflammatory diet. Topped with a sprinkle of cinnamon and a drizzle of maple syrup, they're as wholesome as they are satisfying.

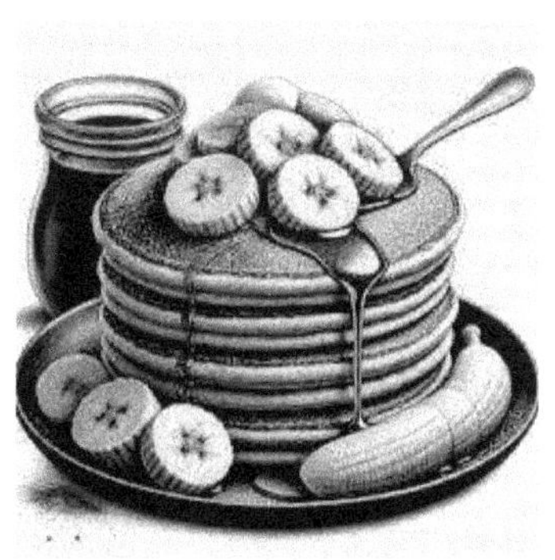

Nutritional Information (Per Serving, Makes 1 Stack of 3 Pancakes):

- Calories: 250
- Protein: 18g
- Fat: 8g
- Carbohydrates: 28g
- Fiber: 4g
- Vitamin C: 10% DV
- Calcium: 8% DV
- Iron: 10% DV

Ingredients:

- 1 ripe banana (mashed)
- 2 large eggs
- scoop plant-based protein powder
- ½ teaspoon cinnamon
- teaspoon olive oil or coconut oil (for cooking)
- Optional toppings: sliced bananas, cinnamon, maple syrup

Instructions:

- Prepare Batter: In a bowl, mash the banana and whisk in eggs until smooth. Stir in protein powder and cinnamon.
- Cook Pancakes: Heat oil in a non-stick skillet over medium heat. Pour ¼ cup of batter onto the skillet for each pancake. Cook until bubbles form on the surface, then flip and cook for another minute or until golden.
- Serve: Stack pancakes on a plate and top with sliced bananas, a sprinkle of cinnamon, and a drizzle of maple syrup.

LUNCH AND DINNER RECIPES

Imagine the sun is at its peak, and your day is bustling with activity. You're seeking something quick, nourishing, and satisfying—a meal that fuels you without slowing you down. This is where the art of crafting a quick and easy lunch comes into play, with recipes designed to fit seamlessly into your busy lifestyle while embracing the anti-inflammatory principles we've explored. In this chapter, you will find recipes that are not only swift to prepare but also bursting with flavors and nutrients that support your health goals.

Quinoa and Chickpea Salad with Lemon Vinaigrette

This easy, nutrient-packed quinoa and chickpea salad is a perfect healthy lunch or light dinner. Fluffy quinoa, chickpeas, spinach, and cherry tomatoes are tossed in a zesty lemon vinaigrette for a refreshing and flavorful dish. Makes 4 servings.

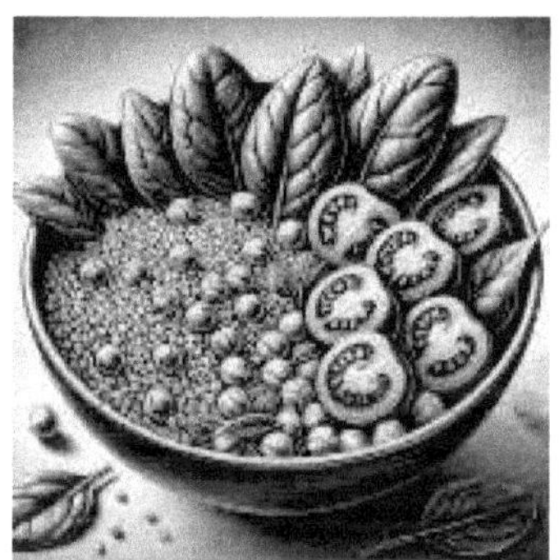

Nutritional Info (Per Serving)

- Calories: 280
- Protein: 10g
- Fat: 12g
- Carbs: 33g Fiber: 8g

Ingredients for the Salad:

- 1 cup cooked quinoa
- 2 can (15 oz) chickpeas, rinsed and drained
- cups baby spinach (chopped if preferred)
- cup cherry tomatoes, halved

For the Lemon Vinaigrette:

- 3 tablespoons olive oil
- 2 tablespoons fresh lemon juice
- teaspoon Dijon mustard
- clove garlic, minced
- ½ teaspoon salt
- ¼ teaspoon black pepper

Instructions

- Cook Quinoa: Rinse 1 cup of quinoa, then cook it with 2 cups of water. Simmer for 15 minutes, fluff with a fork, and let it cool.
- Prep Vegetables: Halve cherry tomatoes, rinse spinach, and set aside rinsed chickpeas. Make
- Dressing: Whisk olive oil, lemon juice, Dijon mustard, garlic, salt, and pepper in a small bowl.
- Assemble Salad: In a large bowl, combine quinoa, chickpeas, spinach, and tomatoes. Drizzle dressing over and toss to coat evenly.
- This bright and hearty salad is ready in no time—perfect for meal prep or a quick, wholesome meal!
- Serve and Enjoy: Serve immediately or chill for 15–30 minutes to let the flavors meld together. This salad keeps well in the refrigerator for up to 3 days.

Enjoy this refreshing and wholesome salad as a standalone dish or pair it with your favorite protein for a heartier meal.

Roasted Vegetable Hummus Wrap

This roasted vegetable hummus wrap combines bold flavors and nutrient-rich ingredients for a satisfying, anti-inflammatory meal. Packed with roasted bell peppers, zucchini, red onions, and a layer of creamy hummus, it's a perfect balance of taste and health. The whole-grain wrap provides wholesome carbs, while hummus adds a creamy texture and plant-based protein. You can personalize this recipe by adding greens or your favorite toppings for an easy lunch or dinner.

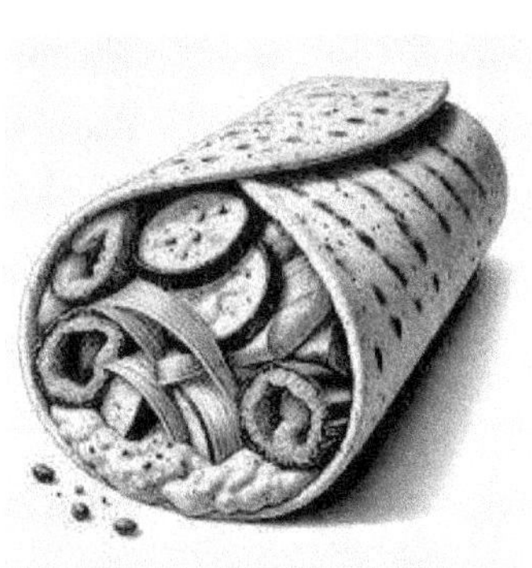

Calories and Nutrients (Per Wrap, Makes 4 Wraps)

- Calories: 320
- Protein: 9g
- Fat: 12g
- Carbohydrates: 42g
- Fiber: 8g
- Vitamin C: 80% DV
- Iron: 15% DV

Ingredients

- 2 bell peppers (red, yellow, or orange), sliced
- medium zucchini, sliced into thin strips
- red onion, cut into wedges
- tablespoons olive oil
- ½ teaspoon smoked paprika
- ½ teaspoon garlic powder
- ½ teaspoon salt

- ¼ teaspoon black pepper
- 4 whole-grain wraps
- 1 cup hummus (store-bought or homemade)
- Optional Additions:
  - Handful of fresh spinach or arugula
  - Sliced avocado Crumbled feta or dairy-free cheese Lemon juice for a zesty kick

Instructions

- Preheat the Oven: Set your oven to 400°F (200°C) and line a baking sheet with parchment paper or foil.
- Toss the vegetables in a mixing bowl with olive oil, smoked paprika, garlic powder, salt, and black pepper. Spread them evenly on the baking sheet. Roast for 20–25 minutes, flipping halfway, until tender and slightly caramelized. Let them cool for 5 minutes.
- Lay out one whole-grain wrap on a clean surface. Spread 2–3 tablespoons of hummus evenly across the center of the wrap.
- Layer the Ingredients
- Serve and Enjoy: Serve immediately or wrap in foil for an on-the-go meal.

This roasted vegetable hummus wrap is perfect for meal prep and can be customized to your taste. Packed with vibrant flavors and nutrients, it's a meal you'll keep coming back to!

Lentil Soup

This hearty vegetable lentil soup is a nourishing blend of anti-inflammatory ingredients designed to soothe and energize. Packed with fiber-rich lentils, fresh vegetables, and spices like turmeric and ginger, this soup offers a delicious way to support your body's natural defenses. Easy to make and loaded with flavor, it's perfect for a cozy lunch or dinner.

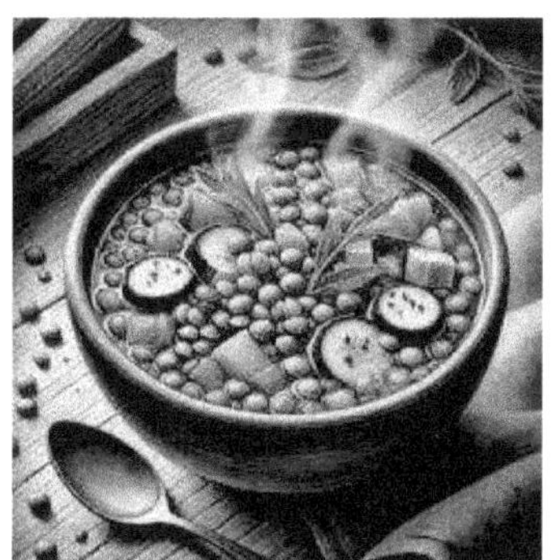

Calories and Nutrients (Per Serving, Makes 6 Servings)

- Calories: 220
- Protein: 12g
- Fat: 4g
- Carbohydrates: 38g
- Fiber: 14g
- Vitamin A: 60% DV
- Iron: 20% DV

Ingredients

- tablespoon olive oil
- 1medium onion, finely chopped
- carrots, diced
- celery stalks, diced
- garlic cloves, minced
- tablespoon fresh ginger, grated
- 1 teaspoon ground turmeric
- 1 teaspoon ground cumin
- 1 teaspoon smoked paprika
- 1 cup dried green or brown lentils, rinsed

- 1 can (14 oz) diced tomatoes (no salt added)
- 6 cups vegetable broth
- 1 cup chopped kale or spinach
- 1 medium zucchini, diced
- 1 teaspoon apple cider vinegar or lemon juice
- Salt and pepper to taste
- Optional garnish: chopped fresh parsley or cilantro

Pre-Heating and Preparation Instructions

- Prepare the Vegetables: Wash and chop all the vegetables. Rinse the lentils under cold water and set aside.
- Heat the Oil: In a large pot or Dutch oven, heat 1 tablespoon of olive oil over medium heat.

Instructions

- Sauté the Aromatics: Add the chopped onion, carrots, and celery to the pot. Cook for 5–7 minutes until softened. Stir in the garlic, ginger, turmeric, cumin, and smoked paprika.
- Cook for 1–2 minutes until fragrant.
- Add Lentils and Liquid: Stir in the lentils, diced tomatoes, and vegetable broth. Bring to a boil, then reduce the heat to low and let it simmer for 20–25 minutes, or until the lentils are tender.
- Add Remaining Vegetables: Stir in the zucchini and kale or spinach. Simmer for another 5–7 minutes until the vegetables are tender.
- Season and Finish: Add apple cider vinegar or lemon juice for a bright finish. Season with salt and pepper to taste.
- Serve and Garnish: Ladle the soup into bowls and garnish with chopped fresh parsley or cilantro if desired.

Tips

- Make it Heartier: Add cooked quinoa or barley for extra bulk. Spice it Up: Include a pinch of cayenne pepper for a spicy kick.
- Storage: This soup keeps well in the refrigerator for up to 4 days or can be frozen for up to 3 months.

This anti-inflammatory vegetable lentil soup is a simple, wholesome way to fuel your body with goodness. Enjoy its comforting flavors and health benefits in every spoonful!

Turmeric Quinoa Buddha Bowl

Fuel your body with this vibrant and nutrient-packed Turmeric Quinoa Buddha Bowl, a perfect harmony of flavors and textures designed to nourish and satisfy. This bowl combines fluffy quinoa, hearty chickpeas, and creamy avocado with the comforting sweetness of roasted sweet potatoes and the crisp freshness of steamed broccoli and spinach. Enhanced by a drizzle of tahini and a hint of zesty lemon, the dish is not only delicious but also rich in anti-inflammatory properties, thanks to the golden touch of turmeric.

Whether you're seeking a quick lunch, a light dinner, or a meal prep favorite, this Buddha bowl delivers a balanced blend of protein, fiber, and healthy fats to keep you energized throughout the day.

Nutritional Information (Per Serving, Serves 2):

- Calories: 420
- Protein: 14g
- Fat: 20g
- Carbohydrates: 48g
- Fiber: 11g
- Vitamin A: 120% DV
- Vitamin C: 70% DV
- Iron: 25% DV
- Calcium: 15% DV

Ingredients:

- cup cooked quinoa
- ½ cup roasted sweet potatoes (cubed)
- ½cup steamed broccoli florets
- ½ cup chickpeas (rinsed and drained)
- cup fresh spinach leaves
- ½ avocado (sliced)

- ¼ teaspoon ground turmeric
- 1 tablespoons tahini
- Juice of ½ lemon
- Pinch of salt and black pepper

Instructions:

- In a bowl, layer the quinoa as the base.
- Arrange roasted sweet potatoes, steamed broccoli, chickpeas, spinach, and avocado slices on top.
- Drizzle with tahini and squeeze lemon juice over the bowl.
- Sprinkle with turmeric, salt, and pepper before serving.

Salmon and Avocado Wrap

The Salmon and Avocado Wrap is a quick and flavorful way to power through your day while supporting your body's fight against inflammation. Packed with omega-3 fatty acids from the salmon, creamy avocado for healthy fats, and nutrient-dense spinach, this wrap provides a wholesome blend of flavors and textures. The addition of hummus adds a protein boost and a hint of Mediterranean flair, while cucumber ribbons lend a refreshing crunch. Wrapped in a fiber- rich whole-grain tortilla, this meal is as portable as it is satisfying.

Perfect for lunch on the go or a light dinner, this wrap is a delicious reminder that eating healthy doesn't have to be complicated.

Nutritional Information (Per Serving, Makes 1 Wrap):

- Calories: 350
- Protein: 20g
- Fat: 18g
- Carbohydrates: 30g
- Fiber: 7g
- Vitamin A: 60% DV
- Vitamin C: 25% DV
- Iron: 15% DV
- Calcium: 8% DV

Ingredients:

- 1 whole-grain wrap
- 3 ounces smoked or baked salmon
- ½ avocado (sliced)
- 1 cup baby spinach
- ½ cucumber (sliced into ribbons)
- 2 tablespoons hummus

Instructions:

- Spread the hummus evenly over the whole-grain wrap. Layer the salmon, avocado slices, spinach, and cucumber ribbons.
- Roll the wrap tightly and slice it in half for easy handling.

Mediterranean Chickpea Salad

Transport your taste buds to the sunny shores of the Mediterranean with this refreshing Mediterranean Chickpea Salad. Bursting with vibrant flavors and wholesome ingredients, this dish is a celebration of simplicity and nutrition. Protein-packed chickpeas, crisp cucumbers, juicy cherry tomatoes, and tangy Kalamata olives come together in 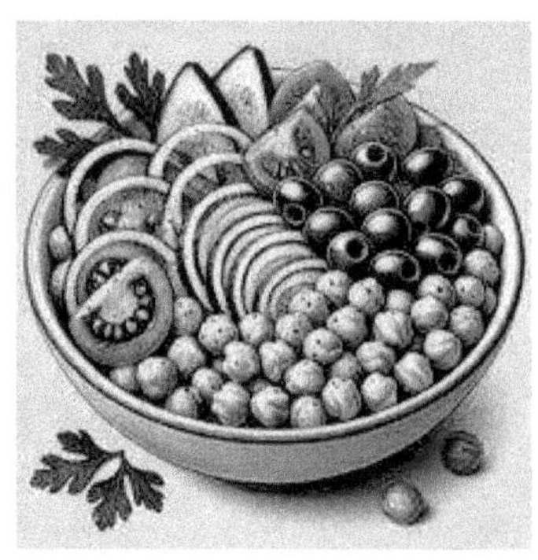 perfect harmony, enhanced by a zesty lemon-oregano dressing. Fresh parsley adds a pop of brightness, while red onion provides a subtle crunch, making this salad as satisfying as it is flavorful.

Ideal as a light lunch, a side dish, or a make-ahead meal for busy days, this salad supports your anti-inflammatory goals while keeping you energized and nourished.

Nutritional Information (Per Serving, Makes 4 Servings):

- Calories: 220
- Protein: 7g
- Fat: 10g
- Carbohydrates: 26g
- Fiber: 6g
- Vitamin A: 10% DV
- Vitamin C: 30% DV
- Iron: 15% DV
- Calcium: 6% DV

Ingredients:

- 1 can (15 oz) chickpeas (rinsed and drained)
- 1 cup diced cucumber

- 1 cup cherry tomatoes (halved)
- ¼ cup diced red onion
- ¼ cup Kalamata olives (sliced)
- 2 tablespoons chopped fresh parsley

Dressing:

- 2 tablespoons olive oil
- tablespoon fresh lemon juice
- clove garlic (minced)
- ½ teaspoon dried oregano
- Pinch of salt and black pepper

Instructions:

- In a large bowl, combine chickpeas, cucumber, cherry tomatoes, red onion, olives, and parsley.
- In a small bowl, whisk together olive oil, lemon juice, garlic, oregano, salt, and pepper.
- Pour the dressing over the salad and toss to combine.
- Serve immediately or chill for later.

Anti-Inflammatory Veggie Stir-Fry

Revitalize your dinner routine with this colorful and nutrient-packed Anti-Inflammatory Veggie Stir-Fry. A medley of vibrant vegetables— broccoli, bell peppers, snap peas, and carrots— comes to life alongside crispy tofu in a savory sesame ginger sauce. This quick and flavorful stir-fry is loaded with antioxidants, vitamins, and plant-based

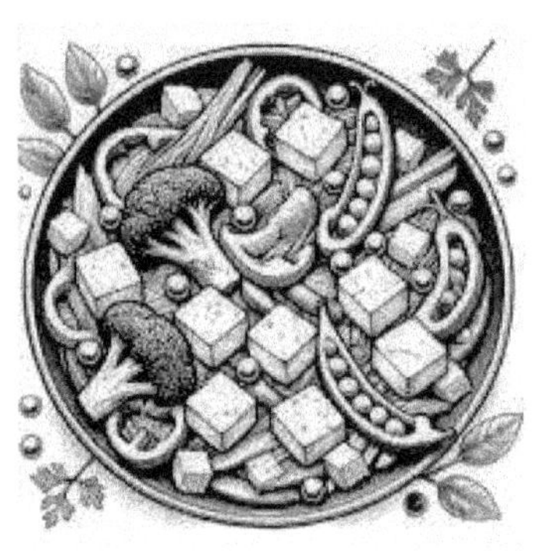

protein, making it a satisfying and health-conscious choice. The coconut aminos and fresh ginger not only enhance the flavor but also provide anti-inflammatory benefits, supporting overall wellness with every bite.

Whether served over brown rice or quinoa, this dish is a versatile, one-pan wonder that's perfect for busy weeknights or meal prep.

Nutritional Information (Per Serving, Makes 4 Servings):

- Calories: 200
- Protein: 10g
- Fat: 9g
- Carbohydrates: 20g
- Fiber: 5g
- Vitamin A: 100% DV
- Vitamin C: 150% DV
- Iron: 10% DV
- Calcium: 15% DV
- cup broccoli florets
- cup sliced bell peppers
- ½ cup snap peas
- ½ cup sliced carrots
- cup tofu (cubed)

- 1 tablespoon sesame oil

Sauce:

- 2 tablespoons coconut aminos
- 1 teaspoon freshly grated ginger
- 1 clove garlic (minced)
- 1 teaspoon sesame seeds

Instructions:

- Heat sesame oil in a skillet over medium-high heat. Add tofu and cook until golden on all sides, about 5 minutes.
- Add broccoli, bell peppers, snap peas, and carrots to the skillet. Stir-fry for 5–7 minutes.
- Mix sauce ingredients and pour over the stir-fry. Cook for an additional 2 minutes.
- Serve over brown rice or quinoa.

Green Detox Smoothie Bowl

Start your day with a refreshing and nutrient-packed Green Detox Smoothie Bowl, designed to fuel your body and fight inflammation. This creamy blend of spinach, banana, avocado, and almond milk provides a powerhouse of vitamins, minerals, and healthy fats to keep you energized and satisfied. Topped with antioxidant-rich blueberries, fiber-packed 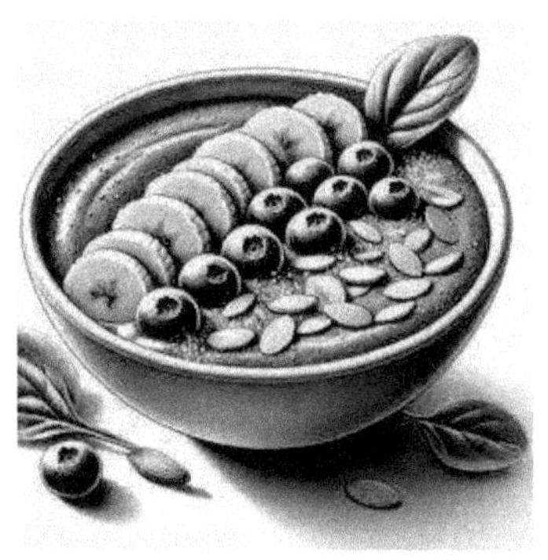 chia seeds, and crunchy sliced almonds, this smoothie bowl transforms breakfast into a delicious, wholesome experience.

Whether you're looking for a quick morning boost or a post-workout recharge, this bowl delivers a perfect balance of flavor and nourishment to support your anti-inflammatory goals.

Nutritional Information (Per Serving, Makes 1 Bowl):

- Calories: 350
- Protein: 15g
- Fat: 18g
- Carbohydrates: 35g
- Fiber: 10g
- Vitamin A: 100% DV
- Vitamin C: 40% DV
- Iron: 20% DV
- Calcium: 20% DV
- 2 cups baby spinach
- 1 frozen banana
- ½ avocado
- 1 cup almond milk
- 1 scoop plant-based protein powder

Toppings:

- ¼ cup blueberries
- 1 teaspoon chia seeds
- 2 tablespoons sliced almonds

Instructions:

- Blend spinach, frozen banana, avocado, almond milk, and protein powder until smooth.
- Pour into a bowl and top with blueberries, chia seeds, and sliced almonds.

Stuffed Sweet Potatoes

Elevate your meal with these wholesome and satisfying Stuffed Sweet Potatoes, a perfect blend of comforting flavors and anti-inflammatory ingredients. The natural sweetness of roasted sweet potatoes pairs beautifully with hearty black beans, juicy diced tomatoes, and creamy avocado. Finished with a sprinkle of fresh cilantro, this dish is a nutrient-dense powerhouse that's as easy to prepare as it is delicious.

Perfect for lunch or dinner, these stuffed sweet potatoes provide a balanced mix of fiber, protein, and healthy fats, making them a fulfilling choice for your anti-inflammatory lifestyle.

Nutritional Information (Per Serving, Makes 2 Servings):

- Calories: 350
- Protein: 10g
- Fat: 12g
- Carbohydrates: 55g
- Fiber: 12g
- Vitamin A: 300% DV
- Vitamin C: 50% DV
- Iron: 15% DV
- Calcium: 10% DV

Ingredients:

- 2 medium sweet potatoes (roasted)
- cup black beans (rinsed and drained)
- 1 cup diced tomatoes
- ½ avocado (sliced)
- 2 tablespoons chopped fresh cilantro

Instructions:

- Slice open roasted sweet potatoes and fluff the insides with a fork.
- Stuff each potato with black beans and diced tomatoes.
- Top with avocado slices and garnish with cilantro.

Zucchini Noodle Salad

Light, refreshing, and bursting with vibrant flavors, this Zucchini Noodle Salad is the perfect balance of nutrition and taste. Featuring spiralized zucchini as a nutrient-packed alternative to traditional pasta, this salad is complemented by juicy cherry tomatoes, crisp carrots, and tender grilled chicken.

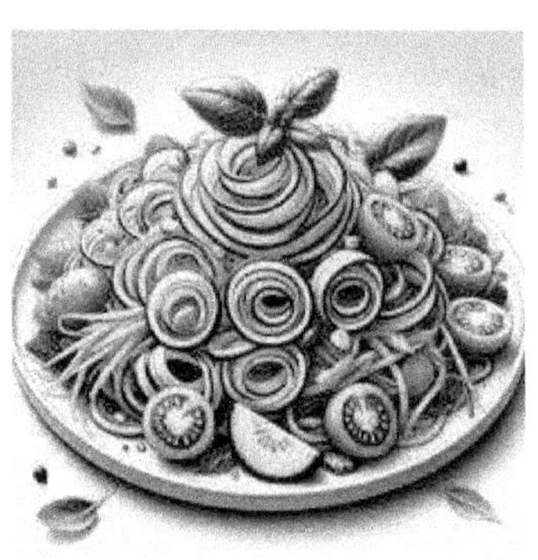

Fresh basil adds a fragrant touch, while a tangy balsamic-Dijon dressing ties everything together.

Ideal for a quick lunch or a light dinner, this dish is packed with anti-inflammatory ingredients that promote wellness and satisfy your hunger without weighing you down.

Nutritional Information (Per Serving, Makes 2 Servings):

- Calories: 280
- Protein: 25g
- Fat: 12g
- Carbohydrates: 15g
- Fiber: 4g
- Vitamin A: 80% DV
- Vitamin C: 50% DV
- Iron: 10% DV
- Calcium: 6% DV

Ingredients:

- 2 cups spiralized zucchini
- cup cherry tomatoes (halved)
- ½ cup shredded carrots

- 1 cup grilled chicken slices
- 2 tablespoons fresh basil (chopped)

Dressing:

- 2 tablespoons olive oil
- tablespoon balsamic vinegar
- teaspoon Dijon mustard

Instructions:

- Toss zucchini noodles, cherry tomatoes, carrots, and grilled chicken in a bowl.
- In a small bowl, whisk olive oil, balsamic vinegar, and Dijon mustard.
- Pour the dressing over the salad and mix well.

Each of these recipes is designed to be quick, easy, and loaded with anti-inflammatory ingredients to support your health while keeping lunch exciting and delicious. Hope you enjoyed eating an anti-inflammatory meal!

Turmeric Coconut Curry with Vegetables

Warm, comforting, and packed with anti-inflammatory ingredients, this Turmeric Coconut Curry with Vegetables is a delightful way to nourish your body and soul. The creamy coconut milk is infused with the earthy flavor of turmeric, paired with fresh ginger and garlic for an aromatic base. Vibrant bell peppers, broccoli, and zucchini bring a medley of colors and nutrients, making this dish as visually appealing as it is delicious.

Perfect for a quick weeknight dinner or meal prep, this curry is a versatile and satisfying choice that can be enjoyed on its own or served over quinoa or rice.

Nutritional Information (Per Serving, Makes 2 Servings):

- Calories: 250
- Protein: 6g
- Fat: 18g
- Carbohydrates: 18g
- Fiber: 5g
- Vitamin A: 60% DV
- Vitamin C: 100% DV
- Iron: 15% DV
- Calcium: 6% DV

Ingredients:

- 1 cup coconut milk
- ½ teaspoon turmeric powder
- 1 teaspoon freshly grated ginger
- 2 cloves garlic, minced
- 1cup diced bell peppers
- 1 cup broccoli florets
- 1 medium zucchini, sliced

- 1 tablespoon olive oil
- Salt and pepper to taste

Instructions:

- Heat olive oil in a large pan. Sauté ginger and garlic until fragrant.
- Add turmeric and coconut milk, stirring to combine.
- Toss in the vegetables and simmer for 10–15 minutes until tender. Season with salt and pepper.
- Serve over cooked quinoa or rice.

Salmon with Lemon Dill Sauce

Indulge in the simple elegance of Salmon with Lemon Dill Sauce, a dish that brings together wholesome ingredients and vibrant flavors to support your anti-inflammatory lifestyle. Tender salmon fillets are pan-seared to perfection and topped with a zesty lemon dill sauce, creating a meal that's both light and satisfying. Packed with omega-3 fatty 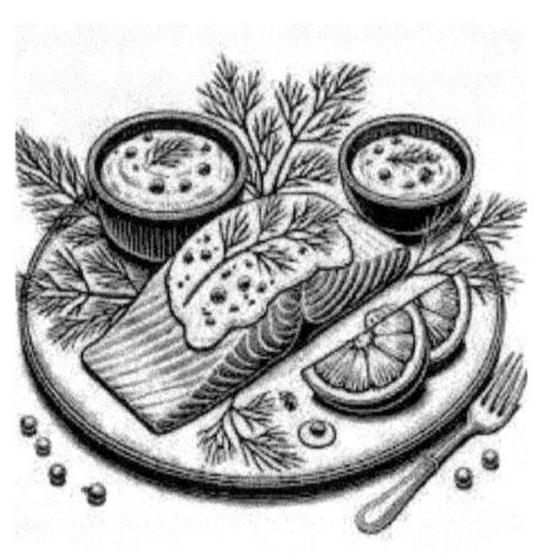 acids, this dish is a powerful ally in reducing inflammation while boosting heart and brain health.

With its quick preparation and minimal ingredients, this salmon recipe is perfect for busy weeknights or as a centerpiece for a special meal.

Nutritional Information (Per Serving, Makes 2 Servings):

- Calories: 320
- Protein: 28g
- Fat: 22g
- Carbohydrates: 2g
- Fiber: 0g
- Vitamin D: 100% DV
- Vitamin B12: 80% DV
- Iron: 6% DV
- Calcium: 4% DV

Ingredients:

- 2 salmon fillets
- 1 tablespoon olive oil

- 2 tablespoons fresh lemon juice
- 1 teaspoon minced garlic
- tablespoon chopped fresh dill Salt and pepper to taste

Instructions:

- Heat olive oil in a skillet over medium heat.
- Sear salmon for 4–5 minutes per side.
- Mix lemon juice, garlic, and dill in a small bowl.
- Drizzle the sauce over the cooked salmon before serving.

Shrimp and Spinach Stir-Fry

Simplicity meets nutrition in this quick and flavorful Shrimp and Spinach Stir-Fry. Juicy, succulent shrimp are sautéed to perfection and paired with vibrant spinach and sweet cherry tomatoes, creating a dish that's both light and satisfying. Infused with the aromatic flavors of garlic, this stir-fry delivers a powerful dose of lean protein, vitamins, and antioxidants to support your anti-inflammatory goals.

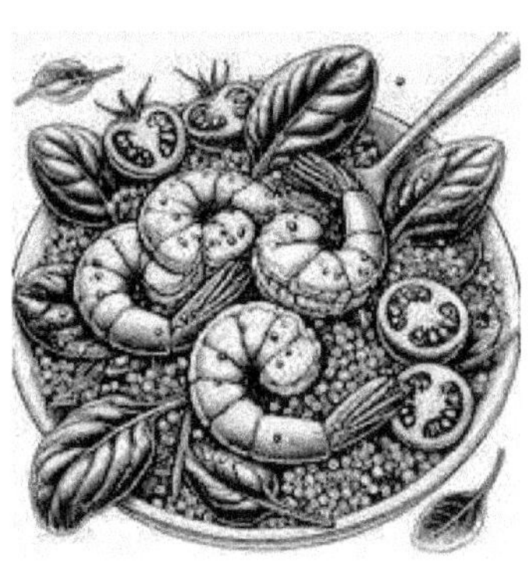

Perfect for busy weeknights, this dish comes together in minutes while offering a wholesome, nutrient-packed meal that's as easy to prepare as it is delicious.

Nutritional Information (Per Serving, Makes 4 Servings):

- Calories: 180
- Protein: 20g
- Fat: 8g
- Carbohydrates: 5g
- Fiber: 2g
- Vitamin A: 70% DV
- Vitamin C: 35% DV
- Iron: 20% DV
- Calcium: 12% DV

Ingredients:

- 1 pound shrimp (peeled and deveined)
- 2 cups fresh spinach

- 1 cup halved cherry tomatoes
- 2 cloves garlic, minced
- 1 tablespoon olive oil

Instructions:

- Heat olive oil in a skillet. Sauté shrimp for 2–3 minutes per side.
- Add garlic and cook for 1 minute.
- Toss in spinach and tomatoes, cooking until spinach wilts.

Grilled Chicken with Avocado Salsa

Light, fresh, and bursting with flavor, this Grilled Chicken with Avocado Salsa is a perfect example of how healthy eating can be both simple and satisfying. Juicy, perfectly grilled chicken breasts are topped with a vibrant salsa made from creamy avocado, tangy lime, and ripe tomatoes. This dish

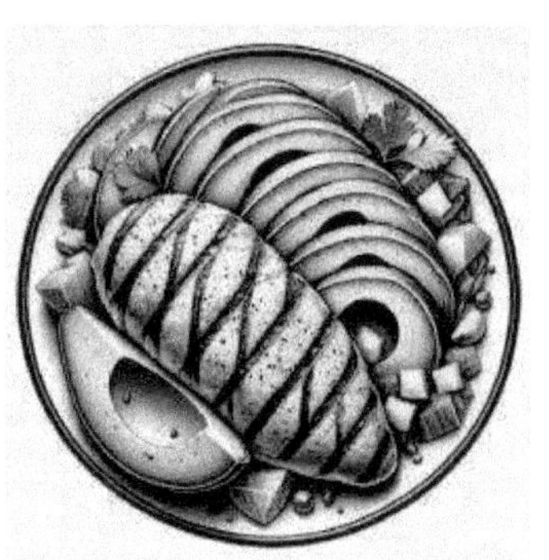

combines lean protein with heart-healthy fats and nutrient-rich produce, making it a balanced meal that's as nourishing as it is delicious.

Whether served for lunch or dinner, this quick recipe supports your anti-inflammatory goals while satisfying your taste buds with every bite.

Nutritional Information (Per Serving, Makes 2 Servings):

- Calories: 320
- Protein: 30g
- Fat: 18g
- Carbohydrates: 7g
- Fiber: 4g
- Vitamin A: 10% DV
- Vitamin C: 25% DV
- Iron: 8% DV
- Calcium: 4% DV

Ingredients:

- 2 chicken breasts
- avocado (diced)
- ½ cup diced tomatoes
- tablespoon lime juice

- 1 tablespoon olive oil

Instructions:

- Grill chicken for 6–8 minutes per side.
- Mix avocado, tomatoes, and lime juice for salsa.
- Serve over chicken.

Sweet Potato and Black Bean Tacos

Elevate your taco night with these flavorful and nutrient-packed Sweet Potato and Black Bean Tacos, a wholesome twist on a beloved classic. Roasted sweet potatoes, rich in vitamins and antioxidants, pair perfectly with protein-packed black beans and creamy avocado slices, creating a balanced and satisfying meal. Wrapped in warm corn tortillas, this dish is not only 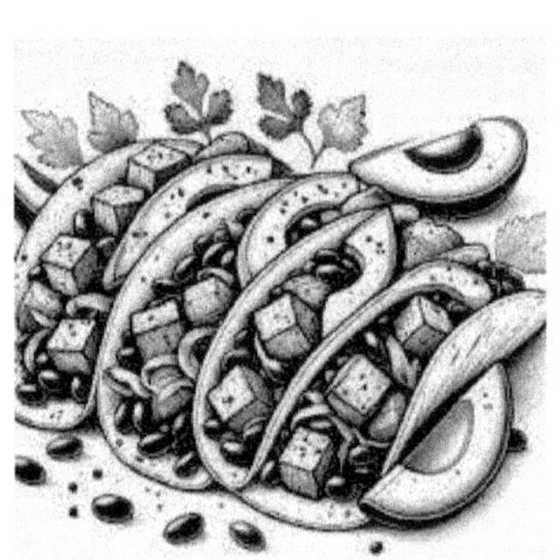 delicious but also brimming with anti-inflammatory benefits.

Quick, easy, and ideal for busy weeknights, these tacos are a vibrant way to nourish your body while enjoying bold, comforting flavors.

Nutritional Information (Per Serving, Makes 4 Tacos):

- Calories: 250
- Protein: 7g
- Fat: 8g
- Carbohydrates: 38g
- Fiber: 9g
- Vitamin A: 200% DV
- Vitamin C: 15% DV
- Iron: 10% DV
- Calcium: 6% DV

Ingredients:

- 2 medium sweet potatoes (roasted)
- cup black beans (rinsed and drained)
- 4 corn tortillas

- ½ avocado (sliced)

Instructions:

- Mash roasted sweet potatoes and spread on tortillas.
- Top with black beans and avocado slices.

Garlic Lemon Cod

Simple yet elegant, this Garlic Lemon Cod is a light and flavorful dish perfect for supporting an anti-inflammatory lifestyle. Tender cod fillets are pan-seared to perfection and infused with the bold, aromatic flavors of garlic and zesty lemon juice. With just a few wholesome ingredients, this dish is both quick to prepare and full of nutrients that promote overall wellness.

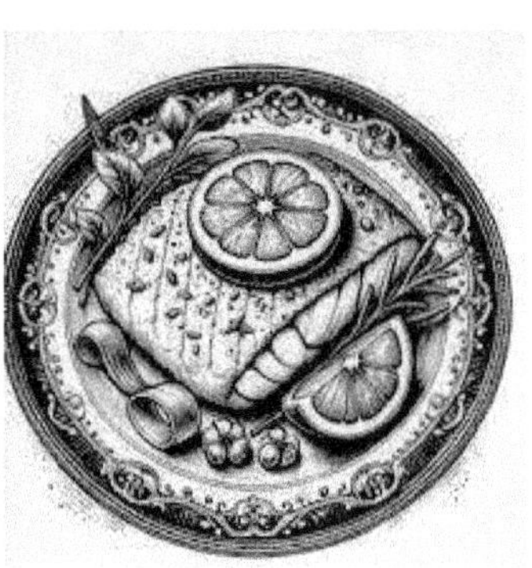

Ideal for a weeknight dinner or a special occasion, this recipe is a versatile and satisfying way to enjoy the benefits of lean protein and anti-inflammatory flavors.

Nutritional Information (Per Serving, Makes 2 Servings):

- Calories: 220
- Protein: 28g
- Fat: 10g
- Carbohydrates: 2g
- Fiber: 0g
- Vitamin D: 100% DV
- Vitamin B12: 90% DV
- Iron: 8% DV
- Calcium: 4% DV

Ingredients:

- 2 cod fillets
- tablespoon olive oil

- teaspoon minced garlic
- 1 tablespoon lemon juice

Instructions:

- Sear cod in olive oil for 4 minutes per side.
- Add garlic and lemon juice. Cook for another minute.

Chickpea and Spinach Curry

Cozy up with a bowl of Chickpea and Spinach Curry, a comforting dish that blends rich flavors with nutrient-packed ingredients. Creamy coconut milk and aromatic curry powder form the base for tender chickpeas and vibrant spinach, creating a meal that's both satisfying and packed with anti-inflammatory properties. Simple to make and bursting with flavor, this curry is perfect for a quick dinner or a meal-prep favorite.

With its balance of plant-based protein, healthy fats, and greens, this dish is a delicious and nourishing way to support your wellness journey.

Nutritional Information (Per Serving, Makes 2 Servings):

- Calories: 290
- Protein: 9g
- Fat: 16g
- Carbohydrates: 30g
- Fiber: 8g
- Vitamin A: 80% DV
- Vitamin C: 40% DV
- Iron: 20% DV
- Calcium: 10% DV

Ingredients:

- 1 can (15 oz) chickpeas

- 2 cups fresh spinach

- 1 cup coconut milk
- 1 teaspoon curry powder

Instructions:

- Heat coconut milk with curry powder.
- Add chickpeas and spinach. Simmer for 10 minutes.

Eggplant and Tomato Pasta

Delight in the simplicity of Eggplant and Tomato Pasta, a wholesome dish that brings together fresh, vibrant ingredients for a meal that's both satisfying and anti-inflammatory. Gluten-free pasta serves as the perfect base for sautéed eggplant and sweet cherry tomatoes, infused with the rich

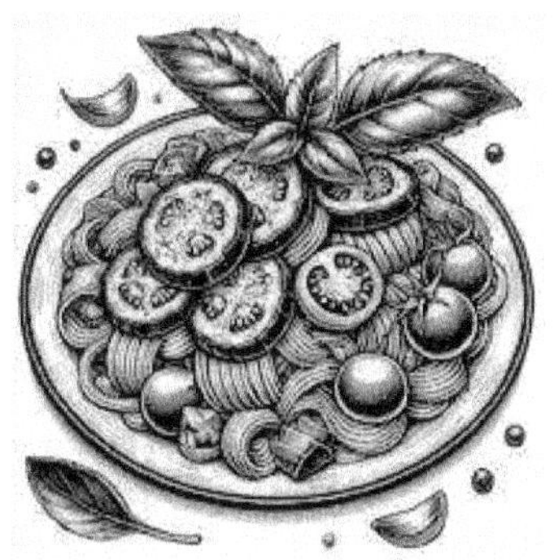

flavor of olive oil. This quick and easy recipe is as comforting as it is nutritious, offering a balance of fiber, antioxidants, and heart-healthy fats.

Perfect for a light dinner or a quick lunch, this pasta dish is a flavorful way to enjoy healthy eating without compromising on taste.

Nutritional Information (Per Serving, Makes 2 Servings):

- Calories: 280
- Protein: 6g
- Fat: 8g
- Carbohydrates: 45g
- Fiber: 5g
- Vitamin A: 10% DV
- Vitamin C: 35% DV
- Iron: 12% DV
- Calcium: 6% DV

Ingredients:

- 1 cup cooked gluten-free pasta
- 1 cup diced eggplant
- 1 cup cherry tomatoes
- 1 tablespoon olive oil

Instructions:

- Sauté eggplant and tomatoes in olive oil.
- Toss with pasta.

Avocado and Kale Salad with Grilled Chicken

Fresh, hearty, and loaded with anti-inflammatory ingredients, this Avocado and Kale Salad with Grilled Chicken is a balanced meal that nourishes your body and satisfies your taste buds.

Tender kale, massaged with olive oil and lemon juice, provides a nutrient-dense base, while creamy avocado and lean grilled chicken add a perfect blend of healthy fats and protein.

Whether you're looking for a quick lunch or a light dinner, this salad is a flavorful and wholesome way to support your wellness goals.

Nutritional Information (Per Serving, Makes 2 Servings):

- Calories: 320
- Protein: 30g
- Fat: 18g
- Carbohydrates: 6g
- Fiber: 4g
- Vitamin A: 150% DV
- Vitamin C: 80% DV
- Iron: 15% DV
- Calcium: 10% DV

Ingredients:

- 2 cups chopped kale
- 1 grilled chicken breast (sliced)
- ½ avocado (sliced)

Instructions:

- Massage kale with olive oil and lemon juice.
- Top with chicken and avocado.

Stuffed Bell Peppers

Colorful, hearty, and nutrient-packed, these Stuffed Bell Peppers are a delightful way to enjoy a balanced meal while supporting your anti-inflammatory goals. Sweet, tender bell peppers serve as the perfect vessel for a filling of protein-rich black beans and fluffy quinoa, creating a dish that's both satisfying and easy to prepare. 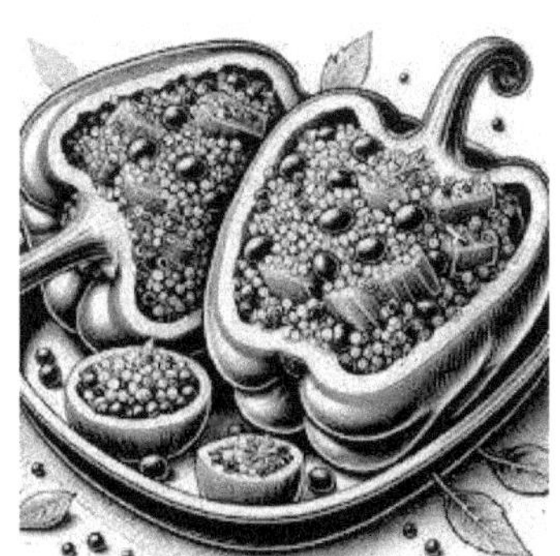

Perfect for a quick dinner or meal prep, this recipe offers a flavorful blend of wholesome ingredients that promote wellness and keep you feeling great.

Nutritional Information (Per Serving, Makes 4 Halves):

- Calories: 210
- Protein: 8g
- Fat: 3g
- Carbohydrates: 38g
- Fiber: 8g
- Vitamin A: 80% DV
- Vitamin C: 150% DV
- Iron: 10% DV
- Calcium: 5% DV

Ingredients:

- 2 bell peppers (halved)
- cup cooked quinoa
- ½ cup black beans

Instructions:

- Fill peppers with quinoa and black beans.
- Bake for 15 minutes.

Broccoli and Turmeric Stir-Fry

Colorful, hearty, and nutrient-packed, these Stuffed Bell Peppers are a delightful way to enjoy a balanced meal while supporting your anti-inflammatory goals. Sweet, tender bell peppers serve as the perfect vessel for a filling of protein-rich black beans and fluffy quinoa, creating a dish that's both satisfying and easy to prepare.

Perfect for a quick dinner or meal prep, this recipe offers a flavorful blend of wholesome ingredients that promote wellness and keep you feeling great.

Nutritional Information (Per Serving, Makes 4 Halves):

- Calories: 210
- Protein: 8g
- Fat: 3g
- Carbohydrates: 38g
- Fiber: 8g
- Vitamin A: 80% DV
- Vitamin C: 150% DV
- Iron: 10% DV
- Calcium: 5% DV

Ingredients:

- 2 cups broccoli florets
- 1 teaspoon turmeric powder
- 2 tablespoon sesame oil

Instructions:

- Sauté broccoli in sesame oil.
- Add turmeric and stir well.

Asian-Inspired Salmon Bowls

Savor the simplicity and bold flavors of this Asian-Inspired Salmon Bowl, a wholesome dish designed to nourish your body while delighting your taste buds. Tender, perfectly grilled salmon is paired with hearty brown rice and crisp shredded carrots, then drizzled with a touch of sesame oil for a nutty, aromatic finish.

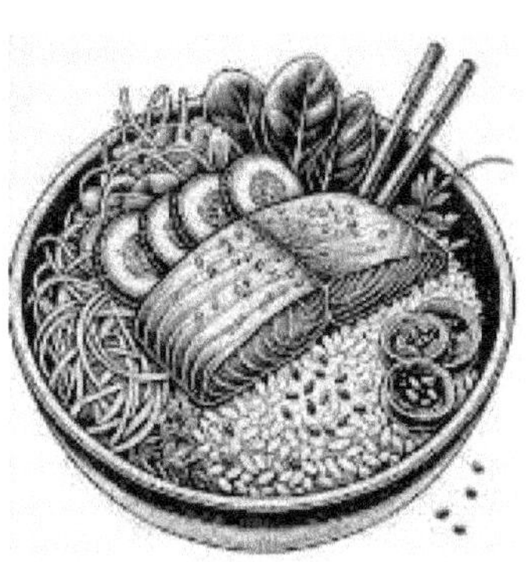

Packed with omega-3s, fiber, and essential nutrients, this bowl is a perfect choice for a quick lunch or dinner that supports an anti-inflammatory lifestyle without sacrificing flavor.

Nutritional Information (Per Serving, Makes 1 Bowl):

- Calories: 420
- Protein: 32g
- Fat: 15g
- Carbohydrates: 40g
- Fiber: 4g
- Vitamin A: 90% DV
- Vitamin C: 10% DV
- Iron: 8% DV
- Calcium: 5% DV

Ingredients:

- 1 grilled salmon fillet
- 1 cup brown rice
- ½ cup shredded carrots

Instructions:

- Serve salmon over rice with carrots.
- Drizzle with sesame oil.

Vegan Cauliflower Tacos

Light, flavorful, and packed with plant-based goodness, these Vegan Cauliflower Tacos are a delicious way to embrace an anti-inflammatory lifestyle. Roasted cauliflower, seasoned to perfection, pairs beautifully with creamy avocado slices, all nestled in soft corn tortillas. This simple yet satisfying recipe is a quick and wholesome option for taco night or a light lunch.

Perfect for those seeking a meat-free meal, these tacos deliver a balance of fiber, healthy fats, and antioxidants to support your wellness journey.

Nutritional Information (Per Serving, Makes 4 Tacos):

- Calories: 220
- Protein: 4g
- Fat: 10g
- Carbohydrates: 30g
- Fiber: 7g
- Vitamin A: 10% DV
- Vitamin C: 70% DV
- Iron: 8% DV
- Calcium: 4% DV

Ingredients:

- cup roasted cauliflower
- 4 corn tortillas
- avocado

Instructions:

- Fill tortillas with cauliflower and sliced avocado.

Greek Salad with Grilled Shrimp

Fresh, vibrant, and full of Mediterranean flavors, this Greek Salad with Grilled Shrimp is a light and satisfying dish that combines wholesome ingredients with a touch of elegance. Juicy grilled shrimp complement the crisp freshness of cherry tomatoes and cucumbers, all brought together with a zesty lemon-olive oil dressing.

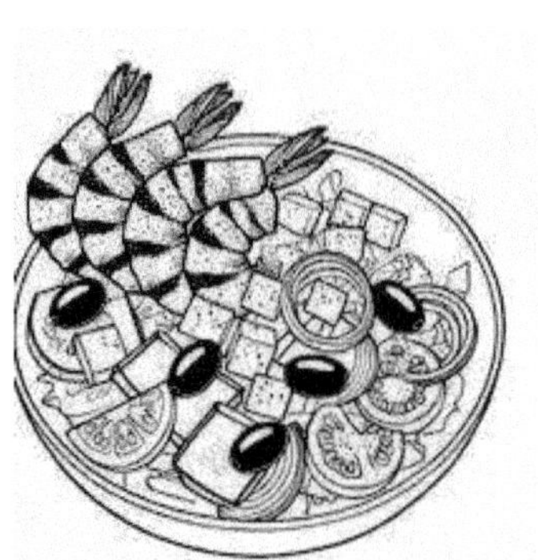

Packed with lean protein, vitamins, and heart-healthy fats, this salad is perfect for lunch or dinner, delivering anti-inflammatory benefits in every bite.

Nutritional Information (Per Serving, Makes 1 Salad):

- Calories: 220
- Protein: 22g
- Fat: 10g
- Carbohydrates: 8g
- Fiber: 2g
- Vitamin A: 20% DV
- Vitamin C: 35% DV
- Iron: 15% DV
- Calcium: 10% DV

Ingredients:

- 1 cup cherry tomatoes
- ½ cup diced cucumbers
- 6 grilled shrimp

Instructions:

- Toss shrimp with veggies and lemon-olive oil dressing.

Lentil and Spinach Salad

Simple, wholesome, and bursting with nutrients, this Lentil and Spinach Salad is a quick and flavorful way to support your anti-inflammatory goals. Protein-packed lentils pair perfectly with fresh, vibrant spinach, creating a satisfying base that's elevated by a tangy balsamic vinaigrette.

Ideal as a light lunch or a side dish, this salad is loaded with fiber, vitamins, and antioxidants, making it as nourishing as it is delicious.

Nutritional Information (Per Serving, Makes 2 Servings):

- Calories: 200
- Protein: 12g
- Fat: 3g
- Carbohydrates: 30g
- Fiber: 12g
- Vitamin A: 50% DV
- Vitamin C: 25% DV
- Iron: 25% DV
- Calcium: 10% DV

Ingredients:

- 1 cup cooked lentils
- 2 cups spinach

Instructions:

- Toss lentils and spinach with balsamic vinaigrette.

Sheet Pan Chicken and Vegetables

When life gets busy, dinner shouldn't add stress. This Sheet Pan Chicken and Vegetables recipe is a quick and easy meal that the whole family will love. Juicy chicken thighs are roasted alongside vibrant vegetables, creating a dish that's both delicious and packed with nutrients.

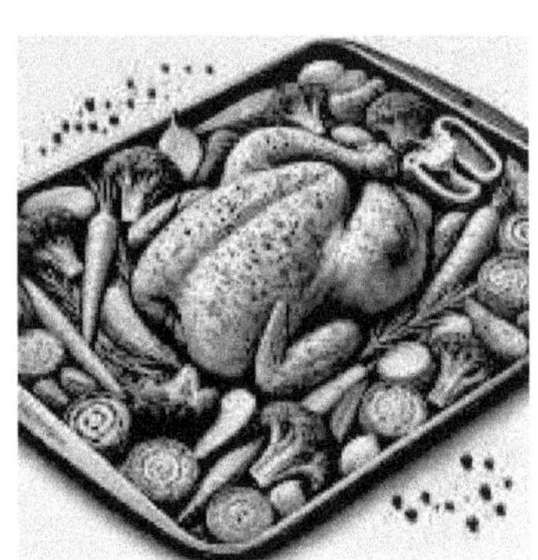

Perfectly balanced and full of flavor, this anti-inflammatory dinner is a win for everyone at the table!

Nutritional Information (Per Serving, Makes 4 Servings):

- Calories: 320
- Protein: 25g
- Fat: 18g
- Carbohydrates: 14g
- Fiber: 4g
- Vitamin A: 80% DV
- Vitamin C: 60% DV
- Iron: 10% DV

Ingredients:

- 4 chicken thighs (bone-in, skin-on or skinless)
- 2 cups broccoli florets
- 1 cup sliced carrots
- 1 cup diced bell peppers
- 2 tablespoons olive oil
- 1 teaspoon turmeric powder

- ½ teaspoon garlic powder
- ½ teaspoon paprika
- Salt and pepper to taste

Instructions:

- Preheat Oven: Preheat your oven to 400°F (200°C). Line a sheet pan with parchment paper.
- Prepare Chicken and Vegetables: Place chicken thighs and vegetables on the sheet pan.
- Season: Drizzle olive oil over the chicken and vegetables. Sprinkle with turmeric, garlic powder, paprika, salt, and pepper. Toss the vegetables to coat evenly.
- Bake: Roast in the oven for 25–30 minutes, or until the chicken reaches an internal temperature of 165°F (74°C) and the vegetables are tender and slightly caramelized. . Serve: Divide the chicken and vegetables onto plates and enjoy warm.

Turkey Meatballs with Zucchini Noodles

This Turkey Meatballs with Zucchini Noodles recipe offers a delicious, family-friendly twist on traditional spaghetti and meatballs. Lean turkey meatballs are paired with fresh zucchini noodles and a light tomato sauce, creating a meal that's high in protein, low in carbs, and packed with anti-inflammatory ingredients. Easy to make and even easier to enjoy, this dish is perfect for a healthy weeknight dinner!

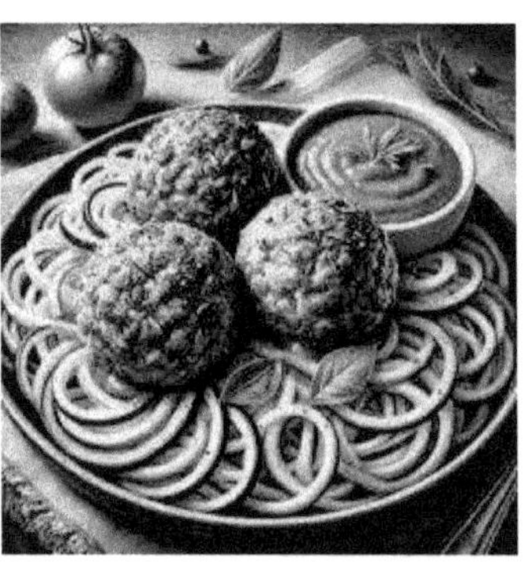

Nutritional Information (Per Serving, Makes 4 Servings):

- Calories: 300
- Protein: 28g
- Fat: 12g
- Carbohydrates: 14g
- Fiber: 4g
- Vitamin A: 25% DV
- Vitamin C: 50% DV
- Iron: 15% DV

Ingredients:

For the Meatballs:
- pound ground turkey
- egg
- ½ cup almond flour
- teaspoon garlic powder
- teaspoon Italian seasoning
- Salt and pepper to taste

For the Zucchini Noodles:

- 4 medium zucchinis (spiralized)
- 1 tablespoon olive oil For the Sauce:
- 2 cup marinara sauce (low-sugar)
- 1 tablespoon chopped fresh basil (for garnish)

Instructions:

- Preheat Oven: Preheat your oven to 375°F (190°C). Line a baking sheet with parchment paper.
- Prepare Meatballs: In a bowl, mix ground turkey, egg, almond flour, garlic powder, Italian seasoning, salt, and pepper. Form into small meatballs and place on the baking sheet.
- Bake Meatballs: Bake meatballs for 20–25 minutes, or until fully cooked.
- Cook Zucchini Noodles: Heat olive oil in a skillet over medium heat. Sauté zucchini noodles for 3–4 minutes until slightly softened.
- Warm Sauce: Heat marinara sauce in a saucepan until warmed through.
- Assemble: Serve the meatballs over zucchini noodles, topped with marinara sauce and fresh basil.

Chicken and Vegetable Quesadillas

Make dinner a hit with the kids by serving these Chicken and

Vegetable Quesadillas! Packed with shredded chicken, melted cheese, and hidden veggies like bell peppers and zucchini, these crispy quesadillas are a sneaky way to add nutrients to a fun and tasty meal. Perfectly customizable, this dish is an anti-inflammatory twist on a kid-friendly classic.

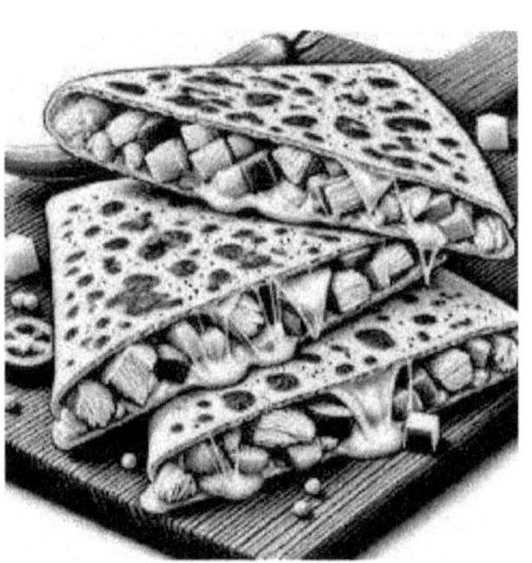

Nutritional Information (Per Serving, Makes 4 Servings):

- Calories: 290
- Protein: 18g
- Fat: 10g
- Carbohydrates: 28g
- Fiber: 4g
- Vitamin A: 25% DV
- Calcium: 15% DV
- Iron: 12%DV

Ingredients:

- 4 whole-grain tortillas
- 1 cup cooked shredded chicken
- ½ cup shredded cheese (dairy-free or regular)
- ½ cup diced bell peppers
- ½ cup grated zucchini
- 1 tablespoon olive oil

Instructions:

- Prepare Filling: In a bowl, mix shredded chicken, diced bell peppers, grated zucchini, and cheese.
- Assemble Quesadillas: Lay a tortilla flat and spread the filling over half of it. Fold the tortilla in half to enclose the filling. Repeat with the remaining tortillas.
- Cook Quesadillas: Heat olive oil in a skillet over medium heat. Cook each quesadilla for 2–3 minutes per side, or until golden brown and crispy.
- Serve: Cut into wedges and serve warm with a side of salsa or guacamole.

Mini Turkey Sliders with Sweet Potato Fries

These Mini Turkey Sliders with Sweet Potato Fries are a delightful dinner option that's perfect for kids and adults alike. Juicy turkey patties served on whole-grain buns with fresh toppings and a side of roasted sweet potato fries make for a fun and balanced meal. Packed with protein, fiber, and healthy carbs, this recipe is as nutritious as it is tasty!

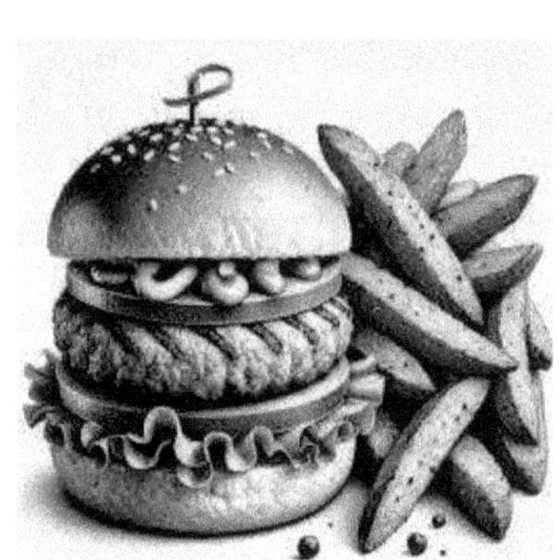

Nutritional Information (Per Serving, Makes 6 Sliders):

- Calories: 360
- Protein: 25g
- Fat: 12g
- Carbohydrates: 36g
- Fiber: 6g
- Vitamin A: 120% DV
- Iron: 15% DV
- Calcium: 10% DV

Ingredients:

For the Sliders:

- 1 pound ground turkey
- 1 egg
- ¼ cup breadcrumbs (optional)
- 1 teaspoon garlic powder
- 1 teaspoon paprika
- Salt and pepper to taste
- 6 whole-grain slider buns
- Lettuce, tomato slices, and ketchup for topping

or the Fries:

- 2 medium sweet potatoes (cut into wedges)
- 1 tablespoon olive oil
- ½ teaspoon paprika
- Salt to taste

Instructions:

- Prepare Fries: Preheat the oven to 400°F (200°C). Toss sweet potato wedges with olive oil, paprika, and salt. Spread on a baking sheet and roast for 25–30 minutes, flipping halfway through.
- Make Turkey Patties: In a bowl, mix ground turkey, egg, breadcrumbs, garlic powder, paprika, salt, and pepper.
- Form into small slider-sized patties.
- Cook Patties: Heat a skillet over medium heat. Cook patties for 4–5 minutes per side or until fully cooked. Assemble Sliders: Place cooked patties on whole-grain buns and top with lettuce, tomato slices, and ketchup. Serve: Plate sliders with a side of sweet potato fries and enjoy warm.

Baked Chicken Tenders with Carrot Sticks and Hummus

Crispy, golden, and oven-baked, these Chicken Tenders with Carrot Sticks and Hummus are a kid-friendly favorite that sneaks in nutrition without compromising on flavor. Perfect for little hands, this simple dinner is packed with protein, fiber, and healthy fats. The creamy hummus pairs perfectly with both the tenders and the fresh, crunchy carrot sticks, making it an instant win for the whole family!

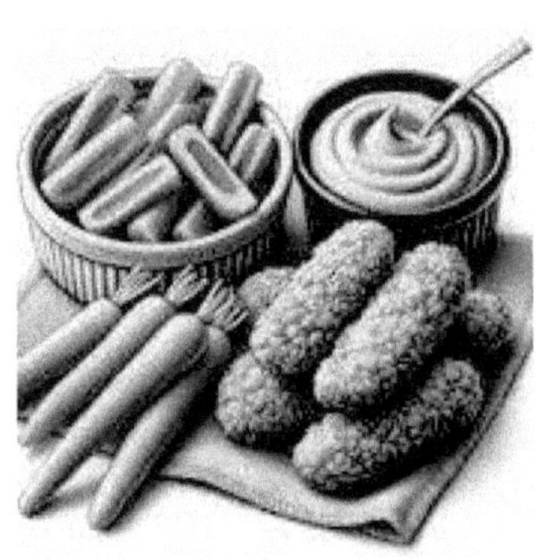

Nutritional Information (Per Serving, Makes 4 Servings):

- Calories: 320
- Protein: 28g
- Fat: 12g
- Carbohydrates: 18g
- Fiber: 4g
- Vitamin A: 80% DV
- Iron: 10% DV
- Calcium: 8% DV

Ingredients:

- For the Chicken Tenders:
- pound chicken breast strips
- cup almond flour or whole-grain breadcrumbs
- teaspoon paprika
- ½ teaspoon garlic powder
- Salt and pepper to taste
- 1 egg (beaten) For the Sides:
- 2 large carrots (cut into sticks)

- ½ cup hummus

Instructions:

- Preheat Oven: Preheat your oven to 375°F (190°C). Line a baking sheet with parchment paper.
- Prepare Chicken Tenders: In a bowl, mix almond flour, paprika, garlic powder, salt, and pepper. Dip chicken strips into the beaten egg, then coat in the almond flour mixture.
- Bake: Arrange coated chicken strips on the baking sheet and bake for 20–25 minutes, flipping halfway through, until golden and cooked through.
- Assemble: Plate the chicken tenders with carrot sticks and a small bowl of hummus for dipping. Serve: Enjoy warm for a wholesome and satisfying dinner.

Veggie-Packed Spaghetti with Marinara Sauce

Transform a classic comfort food into a nutrient-rich, family-friendly dinner with this Veggie-Packed Spaghetti with Marinara Sauce. Loaded with hidden vegetables like zucchini, carrots, and spinach, this dish is a clever way to add vitamins and fiber to a meal kids already love. It's wholesome, satisfying, and quick to prepare—perfect for busy weeknights!

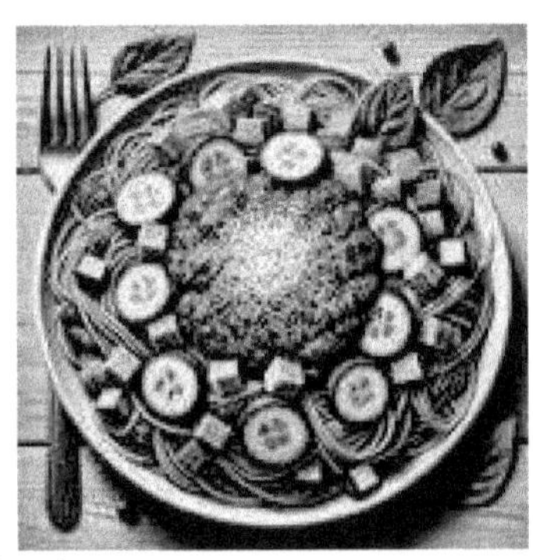

Nutritional Information (Per Serving, Makes 4 Servings):

Calories: 320

Protein: 10g

Fat: 8g

Carbohydrates: 52g

Fiber: 6g

Vitamin A: 80% DV

Vitamin C: 25% DV Iron: 15% DV

Ingredients:

For the Spaghetti:

- 8 ounces whole-grain or gluten-free spaghetti
- 1 cup finely diced carrots
- 1 cup finely diced zucchini
- 1 cup chopped spinach

For the Sauce:

- cups marinara sauce (low-sugar)
- tablespoon olive oil

- Optional: grated Parmesan cheese for topping

Instructions:

- Cook Pasta: Boil spaghetti according to package instructions. Drain and set aside.
- Sauté Vegetables: Heat olive oil in a large skillet over medium heat. Sauté carrots and zucchini for 5 minutes.
- Add spinach and cook until wilted.
- Add Sauce: Stir in marinara sauce and simmer for 3–5 minutes.
- Combine: Toss the cooked spaghetti with the veggie marinara sauce.
- Serve: Plate and sprinkle with grated Parmesan cheese if desired.

Baked Veggie Nuggets

Make veggies irresistible with these Baked Veggie Nuggets, a kid-approved dinner packed with hidden nutrients. These crispy nuggets, made from carrots, broccoli, and cauliflower, are a delightful alternative to traditional options. Perfect for little hands and paired with a side of ketchup and fresh cucumber sticks, this dish is a fun, healthy, and flavorful way to make dinner time exciting.

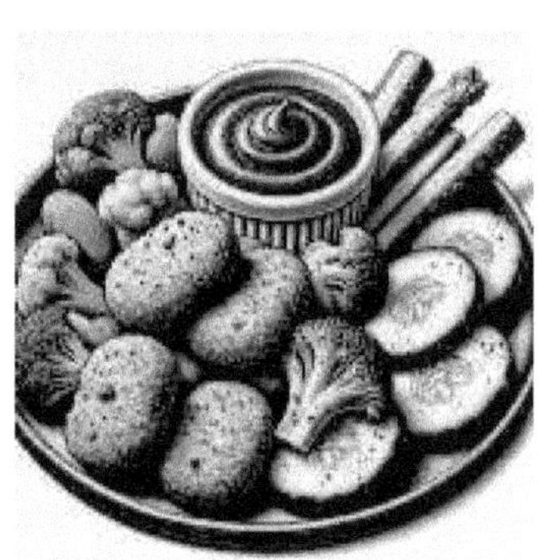

Nutritional Information (Per Serving, Makes 4 Servings):

- Calories: 210
- Protein: 8g
- Fat: 7g
- Carbohydrates: 30g
- Fiber: 6g
- Vitamin A: 120% DV
- Vitamin C: 60% DV
- Iron: 10% DV

Ingredients:

- 1 cup steamed carrots (mashed)
- 1 cup steamed broccoli (chopped)
- 1 cup steamed cauliflower (chopped)
- ½ cup breadcrumbs (gluten-free or regular)
- 1 egg
- ½ teaspoon garlic powder
- Salt and pepper to taste
- 1 tablespoon olive oil (for brushing)
- Ketchup for dipping

- 1 cup cucumber sticks (optional, for serving)

Instructions:

- Preheat Oven: Preheat your oven to 375°F (190°C). Line a baking sheet with parchment paper.
- Mix Ingredients: In a bowl, combine mashed carrots, chopped broccoli, cauliflower, breadcrumbs, egg, garlic powder, salt, and pepper. Mix well.
- Form Nuggets: Shape the mixture into nugget-sized pieces and place them on the baking sheet.
- Bake: Brush the nuggets with olive oil and bake for 20–25 minutes, flipping halfway through, until golden and crispy.
- Serve: Plate the nuggets with a side of ketchup and cucumber sticks for dipping.

Cheesy Cauliflower Mac and Cheese

Comfort food meets wholesome nutrition in this Cheesy

Cauliflower Mac and Cheese. Made with a creamy cauliflower-based sauce and gluten-free pasta, this kid-friendly dish is packed with hidden vegetables and free from artificial ingredients. A sprinkle of breadcrumbs on top adds the

perfect crunch, making it a delightful and nourishing meal the whole family will love.

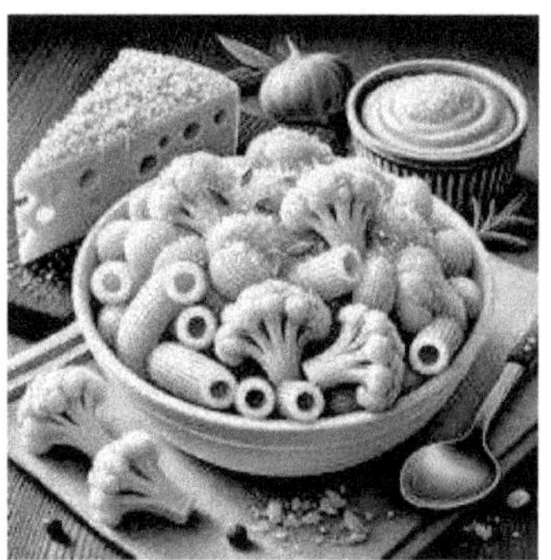

Nutritional Information (Per Serving, Makes 4 Servings):

- Calories: 290
- Protein: 12g
- Fat: 9g
- Carbohydrates: 40g
- Fiber: 6g
- Vitamin C: 30% DV
- Calcium: 15% DV
- Iron: 10% DV

Ingredients:

For the Mac and Cheese:
- 8 ounces gluten-free pasta (elbow or shell-shaped)
- cup steamed cauliflower (mashed) ½ cup shredded cheddar cheese (or dairy-free alternative)
- ½ cup unsweetened almond milk
- 1 teaspoon garlic powder
- Salt and pepper to taste

For the Topping:

- 2 tablespoons gluten-free breadcrumbs
  - 1 teaspoon olive oil

Instructions:

- Cook Pasta: Boil pasta according to package instructions.
- Drain and set aside.
- Prepare Sauce: In a blender or food processor, blend steamed cauliflower, cheddar cheese, almond milk, garlic powder, salt, and pepper until smooth.
- Combine: Mix the pasta with the cauliflower cheese sauce in a large saucepan over medium heat. Stir until heated through.
- Add Topping: In a small skillet, toast breadcrumbs in olive oil until golden. Sprinkle over the mac and cheese before serving.

Mini Veggie Pizzas

Turn dinner into a fun, hands-on experience with these Mini Veggie Pizzas! Using whole-grain English muffins as the base, these customizable pizzas are topped with a medley of colorful vegetables and gooey cheese. They're a perfect way to get kids excited about eating their veggies while enjoying a quick, nutritious meal that's as fun to make as it is to eat.

Nutritional Information (Per Serving, Makes 4 Servings):

- Calories: 230
- Protein: 10g
- Fat: 7g
- Carbohydrates: 28g
- Fiber: 5g
- Vitamin A: 25% DV
- Vitamin C: 40% DV Calcium: 20% DV

Ingredients:

- 4 whole-grain English muffins (halved)
- ½ cup tomato sauce (low-sodium)
- cup shredded mozzarella cheese (or dairy-free alternative)
- ½ cup diced bell peppers
- ½ cup chopped spinach
- ½ cup halved cherry tomatoes

Instructions:

- Preheat Oven: Preheat your oven to 375°F (190°C). Line a baking sheet with parchment paper.

- Assemble Pizzas: Place English muffin halves on the baking sheet. Spread 1 tablespoon of tomato sauce on each half.
- Add Toppings: Sprinkle shredded cheese over the sauce and top with bell peppers, spinach, and cherry tomatoes. Bake: Bake for 10–12 minutes, or until the cheese is melted and bubbly. Serve: Let cool slightly before serving.
- Enjoy warm for a delightful meal!

Cheesy Zucchini Boats

These Cheesy Zucchini Boats are a fun and nutritious dinner that kids will adore! Hollowed-out zucchini halves are stuffed with a cheesy mixture, diced tomatoes, and breadcrumbs, then baked to perfection. This recipe is a clever way to introduce vegetables in a delicious and visually appealing way, making it a great addition to your family-friendly meal rotation.

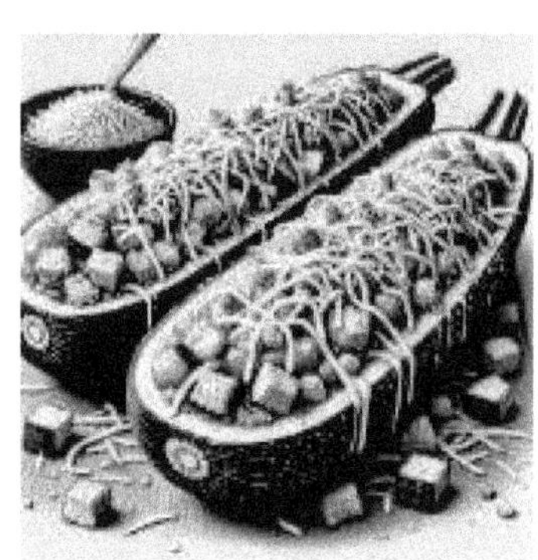

Nutritional Information (Per Serving, Makes 4 Servings):

- Calories: 210
- Protein: 9g
- Fat: 10g
- Carbohydrates: 20g Fiber: 3g
- Vitamin C: 25% DV
- Calcium: 15% DV Iron: 8% DV

Ingredients:

- 2 medium zucchinis (halved lengthwise, seeds removed) ½ cup shredded mozzarella cheese (or dairy-free alternative)
- ½ cup diced tomatoes
- ¼ cup breadcrumbs (gluten-free or regular)
- tablespoon olive oil
- Salt and pepper to taste

Instructions:

- Preheat Oven: Preheat your oven to 375°F (190°C). Line a baking sheet with parchment paper.

- Prepare Zucchini: Scoop out the seeds from the zucchini halves to create a hollow center.
- Stuff the Zucchini: Mix shredded cheese, diced tomatoes, breadcrumbs, salt, and pepper in a bowl. Fill each zucchini half with the mixture.
- Bake: Place the zucchini boats on the baking sheet. Drizzle with olive oil and bake for 20–25 minutes, or until the zucchini is tender and the cheese is melted.
- Serve: Let cool slightly before serving. Enjoy warm as a wholesome main or side dish.

Baked Sweet Potato Fries with Honey Mustard Dip

Transform a simple side into a standout dish with these Baked Sweet Potato Fries with Honey Mustard Dip. Crispy on the edges and tender on the inside, these fries are a delightful, nutrient- packed option for kids and adults alike. Paired with a creamy homemade honey mustard sauce, this dish balances sweet and savory flavors, making it a perfect addition to any family dinner.

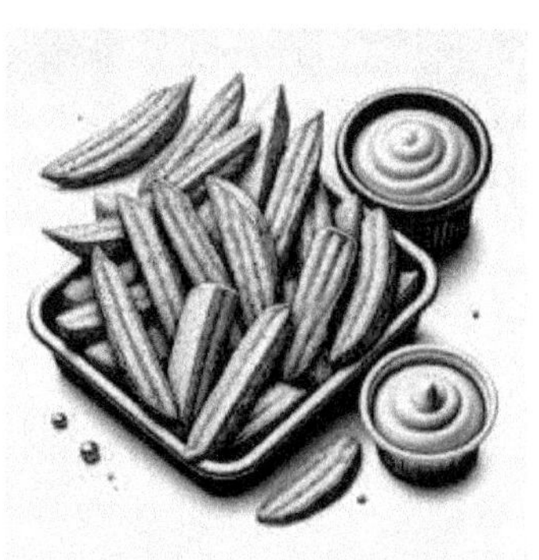

Nutritional Information (Per Serving, Makes 4 Servings):

- Calories: 180
- Protein: 3g
- Fat: 6g
- Carbohydrates: 30g
- Fiber: 5g
- Vitamin A: 200% DV
- Iron: 6% DV
- Calcium: 4% DV

Ingredients:

For the Fries:

- 2 medium sweet potatoes (cut into thin wedges)
- 1 tablespoon olive oil
- ½ teaspoon paprika
- ¼ teaspoon garlic powder
- Salt to taste

For the Honey Mustard Dip:

- 2 tablespoons Greek yogurt
- tablespoon Dijon mustard teaspoon honey

Instructions:

- Preheat Oven: Preheat your oven to 400°F (200°C). Line a baking sheet with parchment paper.
- Prepare Fries: Toss sweet potato wedges with olive oil, paprika, garlic powder, and salt until evenly coated.
- Arrange on the baking sheet in a single layer.
- Bake: Roast for 25–30 minutes, flipping halfway through, until crispy on the edges and tender inside. Make the Dip: In a small bowl, whisk together Greek yogurt, Dijon mustard, and honey until smooth. Serve: Plate the sweet potato fries with a side of honey mustard dip and enjoy warm.

Turkey and Vegetable Meatballs

These Turkey and Vegetable Meatballs are a wholesome and flavorful dinner option that the whole family will enjoy. Packed with lean turkey, finely chopped vegetables, and herbs, these meatballs are tender, juicy, and perfect for dipping in marinara sauce. They're easy to prepare, nutrient-rich, and a fun way to sneak more veggies into your kid's meal.

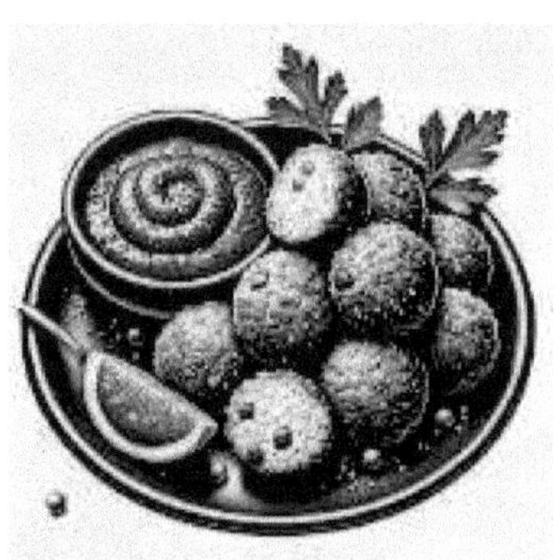

Nutritional Information (Per Serving, Makes 4 Servings):

- Calories: 230
- Protein: 20g
- Fat: 10g
- Carbohydrates: 12g
- Fiber: 2g
- Vitamin A: 30% DV
- Vitamin C: 15% DV Iron: 10% DV

Ingredients:

- pound ground turkey
- cup finely grated zucchini
- ½ cup finely chopped carrots
- egg
- ½ cup breadcrumbs (gluten-free or regular)
- teaspoon garlic powder
- ½ teaspoon paprika
- Salt and pepper to taste
- Marinara sauce for dipping

nstructions:

- Preheat Oven: Preheat your oven to 375°F (190°C). Line a baking sheet with parchment paper.
- Mix Ingredients: In a large bowl, combine ground turkey, zucchini, carrots, egg, breadcrumbs, garlic powder, paprika, salt, and pepper. Mix until well combined. . Form Meatballs: Roll the mixture into 1-inch balls and place them on the prepared baking sheet. Bake: Bake for 20–25 minutes, or until golden brown and cooked through.
- Serve: Plate the meatballs with a side of warm marinara sauce for dipping.

SIMPLE SNACKS AND SMOOTHIES

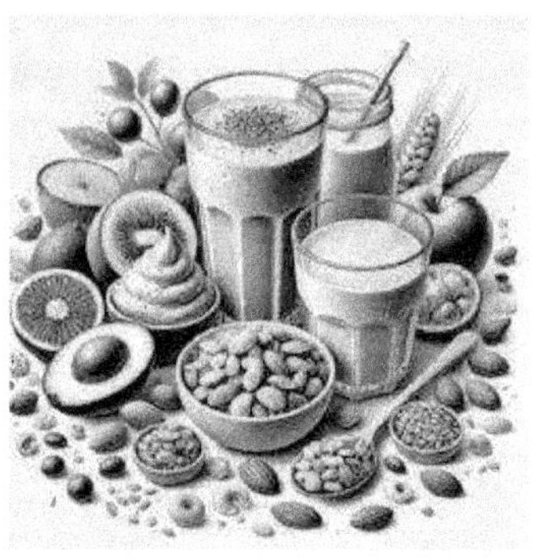

In the midst of your day, when energy levels dip and hunger strikes, having quick and nutritious snacks at hand can make all the difference. A homemade trail mix is a perfect companion, combining the satisfying crunch of nuts with the subtle sweetness of dried fruit. Consider almonds, walnuts, and cashews mingling with dried cranberries and apricots. These ingredients create a balanced snack rich in healthy fats and antioxidants, supporting your body's fight against inflammation while keeping hunger at bay. For a touch of indulgence, add a few dark chocolate chips. This simple mix can be prepared in bulk and portioned out, ready to accompany you throughout the day.

Rice cakes offer another versatile snacking option. Spread a thin layer of almond butter on top, then add banana slices for a naturally sweet and creamy finish. This combination is not just delicious; it also provides a quick energy boost from the carbohydrates in the rice cake and the potassium in the banana. The almond butter adds a dose of healthy fats and protein, helping to regulate blood sugar levels and sustain energy. It's a snack that requires no more than a moment to assemble, yet delivers satisfaction and nourishment that lasts.

Smoothies, with their convenience and adaptability, are ideal for those on the go. A green smoothie featuring spinach, kiwi, and flaxseed is a vibrant choice. Blend these ingredients with a splash of coconut water or almond milk, and you've created a drink that's refreshing and nutrient-dense. Spinach contributes iron and folate, while kiwi adds vitamin C and a zesty sweetness. Flaxseed, REVIVING YOUR BODY WITH THE ANTI-INFLAMMATORY DIE... known for its omega-3 fatty acids, supports heart health and inflammation reduction.

This smoothie is not just a drink but a liquid meal that fuels your body and mind.

For a berry-forward option, a smoothie with Greek yogurt, mixed berries, and a sprinkle of chia seeds offers a symphony of flavors and textures. The tartness of berries, rich in antioxidants, pairs beautifully with the creamy yogurt, which provides probiotics and protein. Chia seeds introduce a delightful crunch and additional fiber, promoting satiety and digestive health. This smoothie can be prepared in minutes and taken with you, perfect for those days when time is scarce but nourishment is essential.

Snacks play a crucial role in managing energy levels throughout the day. They help bridge the gap between meals, preventing the dips in blood sugar that often lead to overeating. By balancing proteins and carbohydrates in your snacks, you can maintain steady energy and focus. Seasonal ingredients add both variety and nutrition to your snacking routine. Think of summer berries blended into smoothies for a burst of flavor, or autumn apples paired with pumpkin seeds for a crunchy, satisfying treat. Embracing what's in season not only supports local agriculture but also ensures you're consuming foods at their peak flavor and nutritional value.

DIVERSE AND DELICIOUS DESSERTS

Spices can elevate desserts to new heights, infusing them with warmth and complexity. Imagine sipping a turmeric spiced chai latte, where the earthiness of turmeric melds with the aromatic spices of chai—cardamom, cloves, and ginger. This drink not only comforts but also harnesses turmeric's anti-inflammatory potential, making it a soothing choice for any time of the day. For a refreshing finish, a ginger and lemon sorbet offers a clean, invigorating taste. The sharpness of ginger and the zest of lemon create a balance that refreshes and delights, while also providing digestive benefits.

When it comes to healthier baking, small substitutions can make a big difference. Swap white flour for almond flour to add a nutty flavor and boost the protein content of your baked goods. Replace butter with coconut oil to retain moisture and add a subtle richness. These alterations not only enhance the nutritional profile of your desserts but also support your body's needs without compromising on taste.

Dark Chocolate Avacao Mouse

Imagine savoring a dessert that not only satisfies your sweet tooth but also aligns with your health goals. Let's start with a dark chocolate avocado mousse—a rich, creamy treat that feels indulgent but comes without guilt.

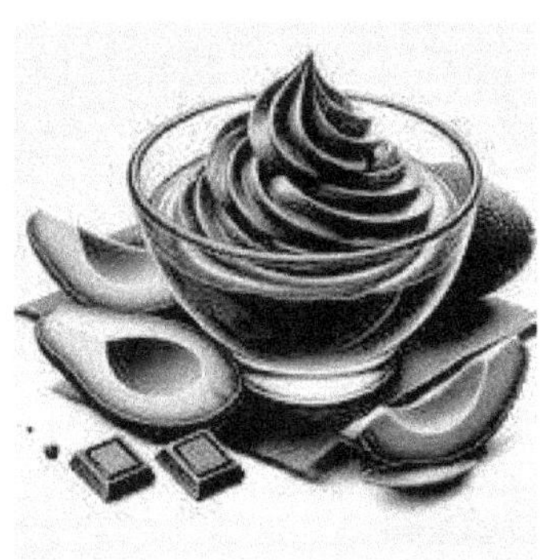

Nutritional Information (Per Serving, Makes 4 Servings):

- Calories: 250
- Protein: 3g Fat: 20g
- Saturated Fat: 6g
- Carbohydrates: 21g
- Sugars: 12g
- Fiber: 6g
- Vitamin A: 4% DV
- Vitamin C: 8% DV
- Iron: 15% DV
- Calcium: 4% DV

Ingredients:

- 2 ripe avocados (peeled and pitted)
- ½ cup dark chocolate (70% cacao or higher), melted
- 3 tablespoons unsweetened cocoa powder
- ¼ cup pure maple syrup (or adjust to taste)
- 1 teaspoon vanilla extract
- Pinch of sea salt
- Optional garnish: fresh berries, shaved dark chocolate, or a sprinkle of sea salt

Instructions:

- Prepare the Base: In a food processor or blender, combine the avocados, melted dark chocolate, cocoa powder, maple syrup, vanilla extract, and sea salt.
- Blend: Process until the mixture is smooth and creamy, scraping down the sides as needed to ensure everything is well incorporated.
- Taste and Adjust: Taste the mousse and adjust sweetness by adding more maple syrup, if desired.
- Chill: Spoon the mousse into serving bowls or glasses. Chill in the refrigerator for at least 1 hour before serving to allow the flavors to meld.
- Serve: Garnish with fresh berries, shaved dark chocolate, or a sprinkle of sea salt, if desired. Enjoy immediately.

Notes:

- Use high-quality dark chocolate for the best flavor and maximum antioxidant benefits.
- This mousse can be stored in the refrigerator for up to 2 days, making it an excellent make- ahead dessert.

Coconut Milk Panna Cotta with Berry Compote

Indulge in the silky elegance of Coconut Milk Panna Cotta with Berry Compote, a dessert that balances creamy coconut milk with the vibrant tang of fresh berries. This refined yet simple dish is naturally sweetened by coconut's subtle flavor, while the berry compote adds a burst of color, flavor, and antioxidants. Perfect for a light, anti-inflammatory treat, this panna cotta is both wholesome and sophisticated.

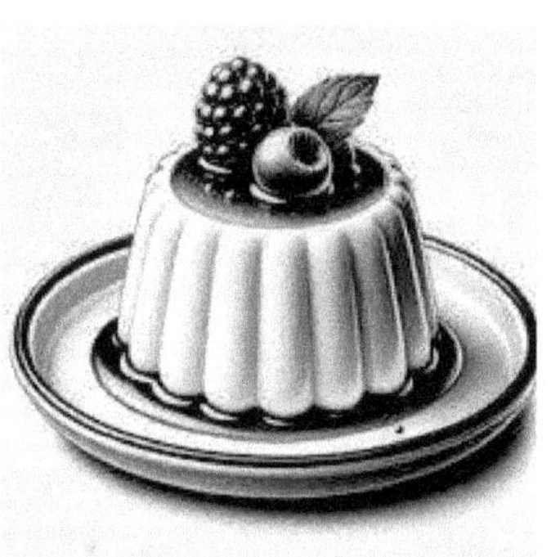

Nutritional Information (Per Serving, Makes 4 Servings):

- Calories: 210
- Protein: 2g
- Fat: 18g
- Saturated Fat: 15g
- Carbohydrates: 12g
- Sugars: 8g
- Fiber: 3g
- Vitamin C: 20% DV
- Iron: 15% DV
- Calcium: 4% DV

Ingredients:

For the Panna Cotta:
- 1 can (14 oz) full-fat coconut milk
- 1 teaspoon vanilla extract
- 2 teaspoons agar-agar powder (or 1 teaspoon gelatin, if not vegan)
- 2 tablespoons pure maple syrup (optional, for added sweetness)

- For the Berry Compote:
- 1 cup mixed fresh or frozen berries (blueberries, raspberries, or strawberries) 1 tablespoon water
- 1 teaspoon lemon juice
- 1 tablespoon pure maple syrup (optional)

Instructions:

Prepare the Panna Cotta:

- Heat the Coconut Milk: In a medium saucepan, combine the coconut milk, vanilla extract, and maple syrup (if using). Heat gently over medium-low heat, stirring frequently.
- Incorporate Agar-Agar: Sprinkle the agar-agar powder over the coconut milk and whisk continuously until completely dissolved, about 2–3 minutes. Bring to a gentle simmer and cook for another 2 minutes.
- Pour into Molds: Remove the mixture from heat and pour it into 4 small ramekins or serving glasses. Allow to cool to room temperature, then refrigerate for at least 2 hours, or until set.

Prepare the Berry Compote:

- Cook the Berries: In a small saucepan, combine the berries, water, lemon juice, and maple syrup (if using). Cook over medium heat, stirring occasionally, until the berries soften and release their juices, about 5 minutes.
- Cool the Compote: Remove from heat and allow the compote to cool to room temperature.
- Serve: Assemble the Dessert: Once the panna cotta has set, spoon the berry compote over each serving. Serve chilled and enjoy!

Notes:

- Adjust sweetness to taste by modifying the amount of maple syrup.
- For a decorative touch, garnish with fresh mint leaves or a sprinkle of shredded coconut. Store leftovers in the refrigerator for up to 2 days.

Date and Nut Energy Balls + Cinnamon Apple Slices with Almond Butter

Indulge in two quick, anti-inflammatory treats that are as nourishing as they are delicious. Date and Nut Energy Balls combine the caramel-like sweetness of dates with crunchy nuts and a hint of cocoa or coconut for a perfect on-the-go snack. Paired with Cinnamon Apple Slices with Almond Butter, these recipes create a harmonious balance of sweetness, warmth, 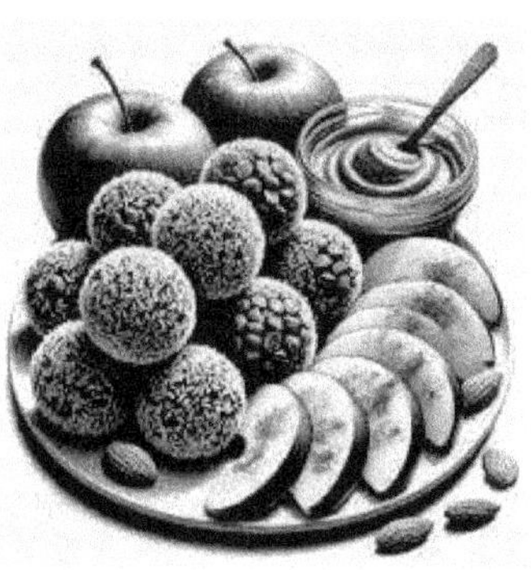 and healthy fats, offering a satisfying and anti-inflammatory boost to your day.

Recipe 1:

Date and Nut Energy Balls Nutritional Information:

Date and Nut Energy Balls (Per Serving, Makes 10 Balls):

- Calories: 120
- Protein: 2g
- Fat: 5g
- Saturated Fat: 1g
- Carbohydrates: 18g
- Sugars: 15g
- Fiber: 3g
- Iron: 4% DV

Ingredients:

- 1 cup pitted Medjool dates
- ½ cup raw almonds or walnuts
- 2 tablespoons cocoa powder (optional)
- 2 tablespoons shredded unsweetened coconut (optional)
- teaspoon vanilla extract Pinch of salt

Instructions:

- Blend Ingredients: In a food processor, combine dates, nuts, cocoa powder (if using), vanilla extract, and salt. Blend until the mixture comes together in a sticky, dough-like consistency.
- Form Balls: Scoop about 1 tablespoon of the mixture and roll it into a ball. Repeat with the remaining mixture. Optional Coating: Roll the energy balls in shredded coconut for an extra layer of flavor.
- Chill: Place the energy balls in the refrigerator for 15–30 minutes to firm up. Store in an airtight container for up to 1 week.

Cinnamon Apple Slices with Almond Butter

Cinnamon Apple Slices with Almond Butter (Per Serving, Makes 1 Serving):

- Calories: 190
- Protein: 4g
- Fat: 8g
- Saturated Fat: 1g
- Carbohydrates: 28g
- Sugars: 19g
- Fiber: 6g
- Vitamin C: 8% DV
- Calcium: 4% DV

Ingredients:

- 1 medium apple (sliced)
- 2 tablespoons almond butter
- ½ teaspoon ground cinnamon

Instructions:

- Prepare Apples: Slice the apple into thin wedges.
- Add Toppings: Dust the apple slices with cinnamon and drizzle almond butter over the top.
- Serve: Arrange on a plate and enjoy immediately.

Dark Chocolate-Dipped Strawberries

Indulge in a guilt-free treat with these Dark Chocolate-Dipped Strawberries. Combining the natural sweetness of ripe strawberries with the rich, bittersweet flavor of dark chocolate, this dessert is as elegant as it is easy to make. Perfect for any occasion, these antioxidant-rich delights are a great way to satisfy your sweet tooth while staying on track with your health goals.

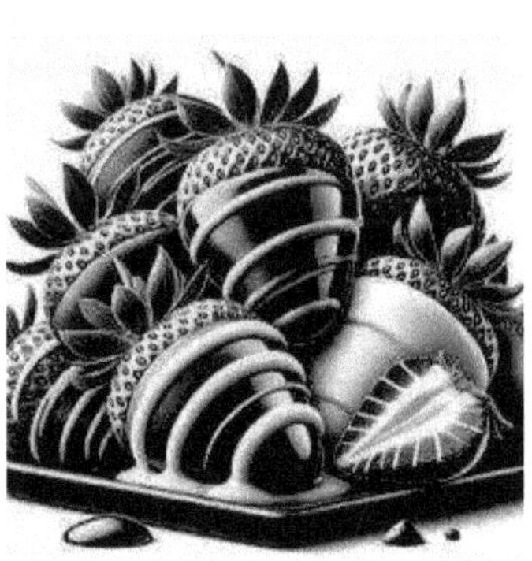

Nutritional Information (Per Serving, Makes 4 Servings):

- Calories: 120
- Protein: 2g
- Fat: 7g
- Carbohydrates: 13g
- Fiber: 4g
- Vitamin C: 50% DV
- Iron: 10% DV

Ingredients:

- 1 pint fresh strawberries (washed and dried)
- ½ cup dark chocolate (70% cocoa or higher, melted)
- Optional: 1 tablespoon crushed nuts or shredded coconut for garnish

Instructions:

- Prepare Strawberries: Ensure the strawberries are completely dry to help the chocolate stick.

- Melt Chocolate: Melt the dark chocolate in a microwave-safe bowl in 20-second intervals, stirring in between, until smooth.
- Dip and Garnish: Dip each strawberry into the melted chocolate, covering about ¾ of the berry. Place on a parchment-lined tray. Sprinkle with nuts or coconut if desired.
- Set: Refrigerate for 15 minutes or until the chocolate hardens.
- Serve: Enjoy fresh or store in an airtight container in the fridge for up to 2 days.

Chia Seed Pudding with Fresh Berries

Elevate your dessert game with this Chia Seed Pudding with Fresh Berries, a healthy and satisfying treat that's perfect for any time of the day. Packed with omega-3s, fiber, and antioxidants, this creamy pudding layered with vibrant berries is a delight for both the palate and the body. It's easy to prepare and makes for an impressive yet nutritious dessert.

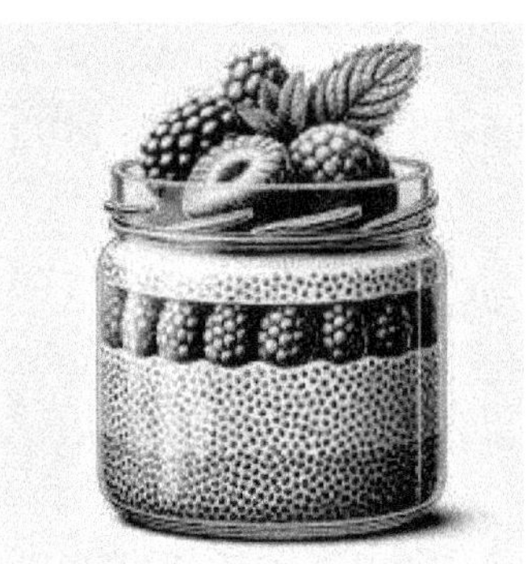

Nutritional Information (Per Serving, Makes 2 Servings):

- Calories: 150
- Protein: 5g
- Fat: 6g
- Carbohydrates: 20g
- Fiber: 8g
- Vitamin C: 15%
- DV Iron: 8% DV

Ingredients:

- 3 tablespoons chia seeds
- cup unsweetened almond milk
- teaspoon vanilla extract
- teaspoon maple syrup (optional)
- ½ cup mixed fresh berries (blueberries, strawberries, raspberries)

Instructions:

- Prepare Pudding Base: In a bowl or jar, combine chia seeds, almond milk, vanilla extract, and maple syrup. Stir well to prevent clumping.
- Chill: Cover and refrigerate for at least 2 hours or overnight until the chia seeds absorb the liquid and form a pudding-like consistency.
- Assemble: Layer the chia pudding in a glass or jar with fresh berries. Repeat layers if desired. Serve: Garnish with a mint leaf or extra berries on top for a refreshing finish.

Banana Nice Cream

Satisfy your ice cream cravings with this guilt-free Banana Nice Cream. Made with just frozen bananas and optional flavorings, this creamy, dairy-free dessert is as healthy as it is delicious. Garnish with a sprinkle of cocoa powder or sliced bananas for an extra treat, and enjoy a refreshing dessert that's naturally sweet and packed with nutrients.

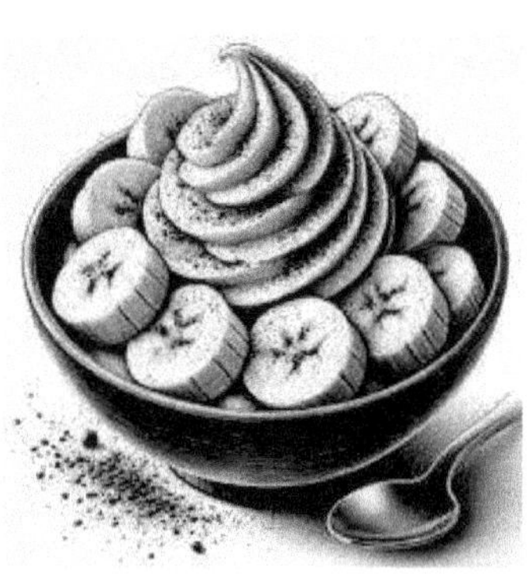

Nutritional Information (Per Serving, Makes 2 Servings):

- Calories: 120
- Protein: 1g
- Fat: 0g
- Carbohydrates: 31g
- Fiber: 3g
- Vitamin C: 15% DV
- Potassium: 15% DV

Ingredients:

- 2 ripe bananas (sliced and frozen)
- 1 teaspoon vanilla extract (optional)
- 1 teaspoon cocoa powder or cinnamon (optional)
- Sliced bananas or nuts for garnish

Instructions:

- Blend Bananas: Place the frozen banana slices in a high-speed blender or food processor. Blend until smooth and creamy, scraping down the sides as needed.

- Add Flavoring: Mix in vanilla extract, cocoa powder, or cinnamon if desired. Blend again briefly.
- Serve: Scoop into bowls and garnish with sliced bananas, nuts, or a sprinkle of cocoa powder. Serve immediately.

Baked Cinnamon Apple Chips

Experience the sweet crunch of Baked Cinnamon Apple Chips, a healthy dessert or snack that's simple and satisfying. Thinly sliced apples are baked to perfection with a dusting of cinnamon, creating a naturally sweet treat that's free from added sugars. Perfect for nibbling on throughout the day, these chips are a nutritious alternative to processed snacks.

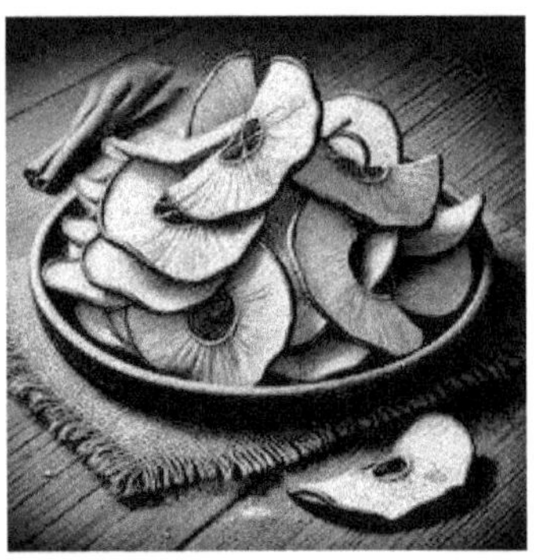

Nutritional Information (Per Serving, Makes 4 Servings):

- Calories: 50
- Protein: 0g
- Fat: 0g
- Carbohydrates: 14g
- Fiber: 3g
- Vitamin C: 6% DV
- Potassium: 4% DV

Ingredients:

- 2 large apples (thinly sliced)
- teaspoon ground cinnamon

Instructions:

- Preheat Oven: Preheat your oven to 200°F (95°C). Line two baking sheets with parchment paper.

- Prepare Apples: Thinly slice apples using a mandoline or knife, removing seeds. Arrange slices in a single layer on the baking sheets.
- Add Cinnamon: Sprinkle cinnamon evenly over the apple slices.
- Bake: Bake for 2–3 hours, flipping halfway through, until the apples are crispy.
- Cool and Serve: Let cool completely before serving or storing in an airtight container.

Mango Coconut Parfait

Treat yourself to a tropical delight with this Mango Coconut Parfait. Layers of creamy coconut yogurt, sweet mango puree, and crunchy granola come together in a refreshing, nutrient-packed dessert. With a burst of natural sweetness and texture in every bite, this parfait is perfect for a quick, healthy dessert or breakfast treat.

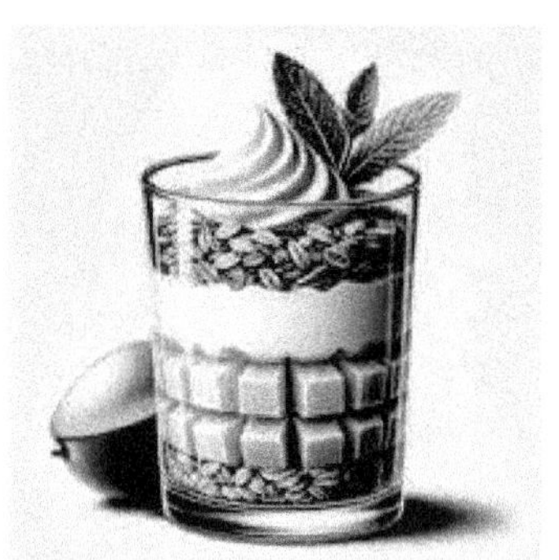

Nutritional Information (Per Serving, Makes 2 Servings):

- Calories: 250
- Protein: 4g
- Fat: 8g
- Carbohydrates: 38g
- Fiber: 3g
- Vitamin C: 50% DV
- Iron: 6% DV

Ingredients:

- 1 cup coconut yogurt
- 1 cup ripe mango chunks (blended into a puree)
- ½ cup granola (gluten-free or regular)
- Optional: Mint leaves or sliced mango for garnish

Instructions:

- Prepare Mango Puree: Blend mango chunks into a smooth puree.
- Layer Ingredients: In a glass or jar, alternate layers of coconut yogurt, mango puree, and granola. Repeat until the glass is full.

- Garnish: Top with a sprig of mint or a slice of fresh mango for an extra touch.
- Serve: Enjoy immediately or refrigerate for up to an hour for a chilled treat.

Baked Pears with Honey and Nuts

Indulge in the natural sweetness of Baked Pears with Honey and Nuts, a wholesome dessert that's simple, elegant, and packed with anti-inflammatory goodness. The soft, caramelized pears are complemented by a drizzle of honey and the crunch of crushed nuts, creating a warm, comforting dish perfect for any occasion.

Nutritional Information (Per Serving, Makes 4 Servings):

- Calories: 130
- Protein: 2g
- Fat: 4g
- Carbohydrates: 25g
- Fiber: 4g
- Vitamin C: 8% DV
- Potassium: 5% DV

Ingredients:

- 2 large pears (halved and cored)
- 1 tablespoon honey
- 2 tablespoons crushed walnuts or pecans
- teaspoon cinnamon (optional)

Instructions:

- Preheat Oven: Preheat your oven to 375°F (190°C).
- Prepare Pears: Place pear halves on a baking dish, cut side up.
- Add Toppings: Drizzle each pear half with honey, sprinkle with crushed nuts, and a dash of cinnamon if desired.

- Bake: Bake for 20–25 minutes, or until pears are soft and slightly golden. Serve: Let cool for a few minutes before serving warm.

As you stand at the threshold of implementing these insights, I encourage you to start small. Begin by making manageable changes to your diet. Try out the recipes we've shared and see what works best for you. Incorporate mindfulness and physical activity into your daily routine. These steps, while seemingly small, can accumulate into significant changes over time.

Reflecting on the personal growth and success stories shared in these pages, I hope you find inspiration. These stories demonstrate the remarkable transformations possible through dedication and informed choices. You, too, have the potential for such positive change.

Visualize your own journey and the healthier, more vibrant life that awaits.

I know that maintaining an anti-inflammatory lifestyle requires sustained effort. Progress can be slow, but it is immensely rewarding. Stay committed to your goals, and remember that every step forward is meaningful. Celebrate your victories, no matter how small, and let them fuel your ongoing journey.

Learning doesn't stop here. I encourage you to continue exploring the world of nutrition and inflammation. Stay informed about the latest research and trends, and seek out additional resources that can enhance your understanding. This knowledge will be your ally in making informed decisions about your health.

I want to express my heartfelt gratitude for joining me on this journey. Your willingness to embark on this path speaks to your commitment to your well-being. I invite you to connect with me and others who share your goals. Engage with our community on social media or other platforms where we can support and learn from each other.

As you look to the future, envision the potential for achieving long-term wellness and vitality. The principles outlined in this book offer a roadmap to a healthier life, where you can thrive and feel empowered. Embrace this vision, and let it guide you toward a future filled with health, happiness, and fulfillment. Thank you for allowing me to be a part of your journey.

REFERENCES

Anti-inflammatory diets - StatPearls. (n.d.). Retrieved from https://www.ncbi.nlm. nih.gov/books/NBK597377/

Anti-inflammatory diet meal plan: 26 healthful recipes. (n.d.). Retrieved from https://www.medicalnewstoday.com/articles/322897

Anti-inflammatory herbs, spices and condiments. (n.d.). Retrieved from https:// www.va.gov/files/2023-09/Anti-Inflammatory%20Herbs%2C%20Spices% 20and%20Condiments.pdf

Cortisol: What it is, function, symptoms & levels. (n.d.). Cleveland Clinic. Retrieved from https://my.clevelandclinic.org/health/articles/22187-cortisol#

Curcumin, inflammation, and chronic diseases: How are they related? (n.d.). Retrieved from https://pmc.ncbi.nlm.nih.gov/articles/PMC6272784/#:

Dietary omega-3 fatty acids aid in the modulation of inflammation. (n.d.). Retrieved from https://pmc.ncbi.nlm.nih.gov/articles/PMC4030645/#:

Emotional eating and how to stop it. (n.d.). HelpGuide. Retrieved from https:// www.helpguide.org/wellness/weight-loss/emotional-eating

Fermented foods can add depth to your diet. (n.d.). Harvard Health Publishing. Retrieved from https://www.health.harvard.edu/staying-healthy/fermentedfoods-can-add-depth-to-your- diet

Foods for fighting inflammation, arthritis and joint pain. (n.d.). Brown Health. Retrieved from https://www.brownhealth.org/be-well/foods-fighting-inflammation-arthritis-and-joint-pain

Foods that fight inflammation. (n.d.). Harvard Health Publishing. Retrieved from https://www.health.harvard.edu/staying-healthy/foods-that-fight-inflammation

Gluten-free and dairy-free diet guide: Health benefits, recipes, and tips. (n.d.). Retrieved from https://www.drbrookestuart.com/gluten-free-and-dairy-freediet/

Healthy eating through the holidays. (n.d.). Harvard Health Publishing. Retrieved from https://www.health.harvard.edu/blog/healthy-eating-through-the-holi days-2018112015386

Inflammation blood tests: ESR, CRP, and PV values. (n.d.). Patient Info. Retrieved from https://patient.info/treatment-medication/blood-tests/blood-tests-todetect-inflammation

Inflammatory responses and inflammation-associated diseases. (n.d.). Retrieved from https://pmc.ncbi.nlm.nih.gov/articles/PMC5805548/#:

Low-glycemic index diet: What's behind the claims? (n.d.). Mayo Clinic. Retrieved from https://www.mayoclinic.org/healthy-lifestyle/nutrition-and-healthyeating/in-depth/low-glycemic-index-diet/art-20048478

Mindful eating: How your food choices affect inflammation. (n.d.). Dr. Catherine. Retrieved from https://drcatherine.com/blogs/womens-wellness/transformyour-health-mindful-eating-and-inflammation

Mindfulness meditation may relieve chronic inflammation. (n.d.). News Wisconsin. Retrieved from https://news.wisc.edu/mindfulness-meditation-may-relievechronic-inflammation/

Omega-3 fatty acids - Health professional fact sheet. (n.d.). NIH ODS. Retrieved from https://ods.od.nih.gov/factsheets/Omega3FattyAcids-HealthProfessional/

Positive reinforcement: What is it and how does it work? (n.d.). Simply Psychology. Retrieved from https://www.simplypsychology.org/positive-reinforcemen t.html

The anti-inflammatory effects of exercise: Mechanisms and implications. (n.d.). Nature. Retrieved from https://www.nature.com/articles/nri3041

The anti-inflammatory lifestyle: From diet to mindfulness. (n.d.). Rupa Health. Retrieved from https://www.rupahealth.com/post/the-anti-inflammatory-life style-from-diet-to-mindfulness

The efficacy of an energy-restricted anti-inflammatory diet on chronic diseases. (n.d.). Retrieved from https://pmc.ncbi.nlm.nih.gov/articles/PMC7700374/

The link between chronic inflammation and weight gain. (n.d.). Retrieved from https://obgynal.com/the-link-between-chronic-inflammation-and-weightgain/

The power of support groups in lifestyle change. (n.d.). Nutrition Studies. Retrieved from https://nutritionstudies.org/the-power-of-support-groups-in-lifestylechange/

The role of nutrition in chronic disease. (n.d.). Retrieved from https://pmc.ncbi.nlm.nih.gov/articles/PMC9921002/

Understanding acute and chronic inflammation. (n.d.). Harvard Health Publishing. Retrieved from https://www.health.harvard.edu/staying-healthy/understanding-acute-and-chronic-inflammation

Yoga for stress: Breath, poses, and meditation to calm the mind. (n.d.). Healthline. Retrieved from https://www.healthline.com/health/fitness/yoga-for-stress